I0407547

Ketosis Diet + Atkins Diet

Special 2-in-1 Books Bundle Edition!

Introduction

I want to thank you and congratulate you for purchasing the book "Ketosis".

This book contains proven steps and strategies on how to lose weight by entering the ketosis state.

Thanks again for purchasing this book, I hope you enjoy it!

This document is geared towards providing exact and reliable information in regards to the topic and issue covered. The publication is sold with the idea that the publisher is not required to render accounting, officially permitted, or otherwise, qualified services. If advice is necessary, legal or professional, a practiced individual in the profession should be ordered.

- From a Declaration of Principles which was accepted and approved equally by a Committee of the American Bar Association and a Committee of Publishers and Associations.

In no way is it legal to reproduce, duplicate, or transmit any part of this document in either electronic means or in printed format. Recording of this publication is strictly prohibited and any storage of this document is not allowed unless with written permission from the publisher. All rights reserved.

The information provided herein is stated to be truthful and consistent, in that any liability, in terms of inattention or otherwise, by any usage or abuse of any policies, processes, or directions contained within is the solitary and utter responsibility of the recipient reader. Under no circumstances will any legal responsibility or blame be held against the publisher for any reparation, damages, or monetary loss due to the information herein, either directly or indirectly.

Respective authors own all copyrights not held by the publisher.

The information herein is offered for informational purposes solely, and is universal as so. The presentation of the information is without contract or any type of guarantee assurance.

Table of Contents

Atkins Diet 164

Part 1 - All About Ketosis

Chapter 1 – What is Ketosis?

Fat, as a dietary component, continues to be the subject of much misinformation and controversy. Many diets, and even diet fads, have emerged in the past thirty years extolling the value, not only of making fat a regular part of the diet, but making it the major component of our daily nutrition. Still, detractors of high-fat diets have called them unsafe and even dangerous, as proponents vowed that going on a high-fat diet is the surest way to fast and safe weight loss, and better overall health.

The Ketogenic Diet has been at the forefront of this diet "revolution," and its popularity continues to increase as new scientific evidence continues to surface and prove that fat does not deserve the bad nutritional rep it has received.

Is fat really bad?

Contrary to popular belief, dietary fat is not bad, but there's a reason behind the misconceptions regarding fat – they are brought by years of misinformation partly sponsored by the US Department of Agriculture.

In the "Dietary Guidelines for America, 2015-2020," issued by the U.S. Department of Agriculture, fats are included in the part where oils are mentioned, stressing that food oils are limited to fat in liquid form at regular room temperatures. The guidelines specifically named vegetable cooking oils, and made it seem like oils were the only source of fat nutrients available for human consumption. Dismissing these "oils" as secretions from fish and plants, the guidelines further pointed out that they do not constitute a separate food group, but exist simply to supply some essential macro nutrients, and on a very limited level, at that.

A "My Plate" diagram from the same USDA report, once again dismisses fat, and shows the "acceptable" five food groups that they recommend being part of the daily diet: (1) fruits, (2) grains, (3) vegetables, (4) protein, and (5) dairy.

The "Plate" includes fruits, grains, and vegetables, and suggests that at least three-fifths of a person's caloric intake should be comprised of foods from these three categories. Incidentally, those categories are foods with high carbohydrate content. Fat is merely mentioned in the context of as oils, which are included as part of food "patterns," instead of being a major food group. Fats from non-aquatic animals, such as beef, pork, and poultry, are not included in the nutritional conversation at all.

However, many recent scientific studies have not only refuted that the exclusion of animal fats from the diet is a good idea. In fact, animal fat is not only an essential component of the human diet, but should be recognized as a major portion of human nutrition, especially when a person is striving to lose weight, and get healthier.

Ketosis

The human body was designed to use fat for energy, and when mostly fat is used for energy, it stores only minimum levels of fat. This results in a lean body, as nature originally designed it, because excessive fat stores are not left inside muscle tissue, "padding" the body. If one goes on a high-fat diet, and the body is starved of carbohydrates, it will burn fat instead of storing it, and during the metabolic process, it produces "ketones." A high-carbohydrate diet on the other hand is more likely to result to weight gain because the body can quickly store carbs that are not used for energy and convert it to fat.

Ketones are molecules that are made in the liver from fatty acids, and are generated from the breakdown of fats. Ketones are formed almost as a defensive action by the body: when the body "senses" that there is not enough sugar or glucose to provide for the body's energy needs, it immediately creates an alternative fuel source.

When dietary carbohydrates are suddenly taken away from the diet, more fatty acids are released from fat cells, which leads to fat being metabolized in our liver. This increased burning of fatty acids in the liver eventually causes ketone bodies to be produced, and induces ketosis, a new metabolic state. Other hormones are likewise affected, and these help transfer the use of this new fuel, instead of carbohydrates, to body tissues. The majority of calories burned by the human body for energy will now come from this fat breakdown.

In short, ketosis is the process where your body burns fat instead of carbohydrates. When the burned fat comes from fat stores, then your body will be leaner, and the chances of having diseases associated with fat and sugar storage will be minimized, or even eliminated.

Getting to a state of ketosis requires ingesting less than 50 grams of carbohydrates per day, so having a fat counter booklet or app on your phone is the best way to start and continue the diet, in order to measure carbohydrate intake accurately.

Chapter 2 – Ketosis Mistakes and Misconceptions

It is useful to know what people, even health professionals, say that might end up scaring you off the Ketogenic diet. There are so many myths and misconceptions that have surrounded, and clouded, ketosis and the Ketogenic diet.

Ketosis Myths and Misconceptions

Myth 1: Carbohydrates are an essential nutrient for good health.

The truth: You can get nutrition and energy from protein and fat.

Myth2: Eating a low-carbohydrate diet can lead to vitamin deficiencies, especially Vitamin C, which comes from carbohydrate-rich sugary fruits and vegetables.

The truth: You can still get vitamins and minerals from some fruits and other food sources

Myth 3: Ketogenic diets cause your body to go into a state of ketosis, which is dangerous.

The truth: Natural ketosis is not harmful to your body. There may be some discomfort at first especially if you're used to a high-carb diet, but it's safe. The misconception is usually brought by lack of understanding of ketosis. Many people mistake ketosis for ketoacidosis, which is an entirely different condition.

Myth 4: Your kidneys will sustain damage from the high protein consumption.

The truth: With a balanced diet, you should not worry about this at all.

Myth 5: A high-fat diet will lead to osteoporosis, because it will cause the body to excrete calcium.

The truth: You can get calcium from sources other than dairy such as seafood and oysters, beans, and bone broth. You can even get it from dark, leafy greens such as kale and broccoli.

Myth 6: Eating fat makes you fat.

The truth: Dietary fat has little to do with body fat. You don't get fat just by eating fat. You become fat when your calorie intake is way higher than your calorie usage

Myth 7: The ketogenic diet leaves out carbohydrates completely.

The truth: You can have up to 50 grams of carbs every day.

Myth 7: Cholesterol from animal fat causes heart disease.

The truth: There is good cholesterol and bad cholesterol. Good cholesterol even reduces your chances of getting certain heart diseases! The ketogenic diet includes food that contains good cholesterol.

Ketosis, of course, means making fat, and to a lesser extent, proteins, a bigger part of the diet. This means relegating carbohydrates to a very minimum intake.

Common Mistakes On Going On the Ketogenic Diet

Because the ketogenic diet is a radical departure from what most people are used to, it is easy to make mistakes. The following are the most common mistakes that can eradicate the benefits of the ketogenic diet, and may even cause harm to your body:

1. To gain the maximum benefits from the diet, you have to be in a state of ketosis for at least two weeks - You CANNOT deviate from this, or you will basically need to start from zero

again, and allow dangerous carbohydrates to assault your system, and create even more fat.

2. Eating too much processed fats and proteins - This is especially true for boxed or TV dinners. While they may have a lot of fat content, there are usually a lot of hidden sugars, and worse, artificial chemicals that can derail your progress. Just because a boxed or frozen meal is high-fat does not necessarily mean is advantageous for someone who is on a ketogenic diet.

3. Eating more protein as opposed to fat - Fat will be your main source of energy, and eating excess protein can actually be harmful, because some of it is converted to sugar.

4. Being afraid of fat - In the dietary world, fat is the friend, and we need to forget all the misconceptions about it.

5. Not getting enough water - Water is the most important element of any diet, and it sometimes helps to give the body a feeling of "fullness."

Chapter 3 – Optimal Foods, Safe Foods and Bad Foods for Ketosis

What we are is what we eat, and this is even more important to remember when one is on the ketogenic diet. It is therefore, very important to know what we can, and what we shouldn't eat.

What to Eat

- Animal Meats: Beef, veal, pork, lamb, goat, venison, and other wild game. Organic and grass-fed cuts are the healthiest options.

- Bacon, pork rinds, and sausage: Make sure that there are no added sugars or excess preservatives.

- Poultry: All kinds, and be liberal with the skin and the fat portions. No need to skim them off anymore. Once again, organic and grass-fed cuts are the healthiest options. Eggs, especially the yolks, are highly recommended. Organic eggs or eggs from grass-fed chickens are preferred.

- Fish of all varieties, with "fattier" varieties, such as tuna, salmon, mackerel, and trout.

- Peanut butter, if very low in carbohydrates, and no sugar content.

- Milk, butter, and cheese (watch out for blends! They may have sugars and other dangerous chemicals)

- Avocados and dried, unsweetened coconuts.

- Non-starchy, green, leafy vegetables, such as leafy greens like bok choy, lettuce, Swiss card, radicchio, endives.

- Kale, kohlrabi, and radish.

- Green asparagus, celery stalk, cucumber, bamboo shoots, zucchini, cucumber, and summer squash.

- Broth, especially self-made bone broth, non-sweet pickles, kimchi, sauerkraut, and mustard.

- Almost all herbs and spices (no sweeteners and preservatives) and recipe enhancers such as lime juice, lemon, and their grated skins.

- Whey protein (keep away from those with sugar, chemical additives, and soy additives.)

- Nuts (make sure there are no sugar-based additives), such as Brazil nuts, hazelnuts, pecans, walnuts, sunflower seeds, sesame and pumpkin seeds, pistachios, pine nuts, and peanuts.

- Coconut oil, lard, olive oil.

Foods that you can eat but only in moderation

- Bell peppers, shallots, tomatoes

- All kinds of cabbage, cauliflower, broccoli, fennel, rutabaga, turnips. Brussels sprouts, eggplant.

- Coconut, olives, and rhubarb

- Peppers, tomatoes, and eggplant

- Winter squash, leeks, garlic, onions, and mushrooms

- Most berry varieties, including strawberries, blackberries, cranberries, raspberries, and blueberries.

What Not to Eat

- Almost all forms of alcohol. Most pure rums, though, have zero carbohydrates

- Rice

- Breads, including wheat bread

- Pancakes and waffles

- Syrups and chocolate toppings

- Desserts

- Breakfast cereals

- Most so called energy bars, including protein bars

- Most energy boost drinks

- Chocolate bars and candies

- Ice cream

- T.V. dinners

- Oils that are processed are generally harmful to the body, and will impede ketogenic progress. These include: margarine, sunflower, cottonseed, safflower, canola, grape seed, soybean, and corn oils.

- Sodas and sugary drinks, and most juice drinks. The basic rule is this: You have to avoid foods and drinks with sugars, carbohydrates, preservatives and chemicals.

Chapter 4 – Ketosis' Overwhelming Success

Weight and fat loss are the objectives of an overwhelming majority of people going on the ketogenic diet. Of course, the associated benefits of a slimmer body can also lead to a decrease in "bad" cholesterol levels, blood pressure, and just better overall, heart health.

Other benefits from a ketogenic have been observed (but not necessarily scientifically proven beyond a reasonable doubt):

- Brain health

- Reduction of symptoms of Parkinson's disease

- Cancer

- Reduction of symptoms of Mitochondrial Disorders

- Reduction of symptoms of Amyotrophic Lateral Sclerosis (ALS, or Lou Gehrig's disease)

- Reduction of symptoms of Epilepsy, especially in younger people

- Improved Focus and Mental Clarity

- Increased Energy

But for weight loss, results are often dramatic and long lasting. Consider the following cases:

"Allison" came from a family of binge eaters, and indulged in binge eating herself. At 230 pounds, she had become desperate, and following the program faithfully, she lost almost 25 pounds after the first month. She managed to stay on track and lost 55 pounds over the nine-month period that she was on the ketogenic diet.

"Tommy" was a morbidly obese diabetic. After going on a high-fat diet, he lost 200 pounds over a period of two years, while hardly even exercising. As he was losing weight using the ketogenic diet, his own diabetes nurse had been a disbelieving witness. Tommy's cholesterol levels, lipid levels, and blood sugar, just kept improving, while eating the exact opposite of the "official" dietary guide we discussed earlier.

There are also those who take the diet in a somewhat light-hearted manner, but also achieve success. "Harry" lost over 65 pounds in 5 months in 2015, and didn't even bother to count calories, much less own a carbohydrate counter. Basically, he ate all the eggs, cheese, meat, and green vegetables he could, while drinking a lot of tea and water. He had moderate success in gaining just a bit of weight during the Christmas season while indulging in sweets, but quickly lost the weight again after getting on a ketogenic diet right after the holidays.

Part 2 – 30-Day Ketosis Plan

The following plan should quickly get you in ketosis after about a two-week period, and keep you deliciously on track for an entire month. I have separated the fat and protein components in the ingredients to highlight their importance in the diet. Good luck!

Day 1

Breakfast

Easy Breakfast Scrambled Eggs (Serves 4)

Fat and protein ingredients:

8 large eggs

1 tablespoon butter

1 cup shredded Cheddar cheese

½ cup diced sugar-free turkey or chicken ham

¼ cup heavy cream

Other Ingredients:

1 teaspoon salt

½ teaspoon black pepper

½ cup chopped onion

⅓ cup chopped red and green peppers

Chopped scallions for garnish (optional)

Directions:

1. In a large mixing bowl, whisk eggs, cream, salt, and black pepper.

2. Melt the butter in a medium skillet over medium heat. Add egg mixture prepared in (1.) and stir.

3. When the eggs begin to scramble, add the ham, onion, and peppers.

4. Continue to stir until eggs are almost cooked. Add the cheddar cheese and stir

Lunch

<u>Sesame Sirloin Salad (Serves 4</u>

Fat and protein ingredients:

2 tablespoons olive oil

One-pound top sirloin, 1 inch thick

Other ingredients:

8 cups salad greens, washed, dried, and torn (radicchio, watercress, and/or escarole)

2 teaspoons freshly milled black pepper

Kosher salt

8 scallions, white part with about 1 inch of green part, cut in 2-inch pieces

2red bell peppers, cored, seeded, cut in half lengthwise, sliced into ribbons

Dressing ingredients:

2 tablespoons soy sauce

2 tablespoons red wine vinegar

2 teaspoons sesame oil

2 teaspoons finely shredded fresh ginger

1 teaspoon kosher salt

Directions:

1. Heat a large skillet over medium-high heat, and then film it with the olive oil. Meanwhile, press pepper into both sides of the meat. Season lightly with kosher salt.

2. Place the meat, scallions, and red pepper in the hot skillet and cook until the vegetables begin to brown (turning as needed) and the steak is medium-rare, about 10 minutes total (3 to 4 minutes per side for the steak). Transfer the cooked meat and vegetables to a cutting board and let it stand about 5 minutes before cutting.

3. Whisk the dressing ingredients in a salad bowl. Add the greens and toss with the dressing. Divide between two large dinner plates.

4. Cut the meat against the grain into very thin slices. Fan the meat over the salad greens and arrange the scallions and peppers alongside.

Dinner

Pork Skewers (Serves 4)

Fat and protein ingredients:

2 lbs. pork shoulder

1 cup virgin olive oil (may be reused later on)

Other ingredients:

Juice from 2 large lemons

2 tablespoons balsamic vinegar

4 tablespoons freshly chopped mint

4 tablespoons freshly chopped oregano

2 teaspoon sea salt

Dash of freshly ground black pepper

4 skewers

Directions:

1. For the marinade, wash the mint and oregano and drain thoroughly. Chop the herbs and preserve these apart in a small bowl.

2. Cube the pork into big cubes. Place these it in a medium bowl and pour the olive oil throughout it.

3. Add the chopped herbs and season with balsamic vinegar. Season with salt and freshly floor black pepper to taste.

4. Combine all of the ingredients, and ensure the meat is submerged in oil. Let

Let it sit in the fridge for 8 to 12 hours.

5. When the meat is marinated, use the grill to preheat the oven to 450 degrees. Note that the meat will barely change color after you take it out of the fridge. This is normal.

6. Skewer the meat pieces in four skewer sticks place them on a rack and within the oven.

7. After about 10 minutes, flip the skewers, and cook until done.

Day 2

Breakfast

Cream Cheese Pancakes (Serves 4)

Fat and protein ingredients:

4 eggs

4 oz. cream cheese

Other ingredients:

1 tablespoon cinnamon

2 tablespoon coconut flour

1 packet of Stevia in the Raw

Directions:

1.   Combine all the ingredients in a mixing bowl until consistency is smooth.

2. Heat up a non-stick pan or skillet on medium high, and coat it with butter or coconut oil'

3. Pour the batter as if it was regular pancake batter.

4. Cook on one side most of the way before flipping.

5. Top with butter, and/or sugar-free syrup

Lunch

Quick Lunch Greens (Makes 4 servings)

Fat and protein ingredients:

¼ cup flaxseed oil (or pumpkin oil)

Other ingredients:

4 cups iceberg lettuce

2 cup rocket (arugula)

4 cups young leaf lettuce

1 small crimson onion

4 teaspoon sunflower seeds

4 teaspoon pumpkin seeds

4 teaspoon sesame seeds

4 teaspoon flaxseed

Juice from 2 limes

Directions:

1. Wash all of the greens and drain them nicely. Tear them in smaller items and put in a salad bowl.

2. Chop the onion into skinny rings and unfold evenly over the greens.

3. Add blended seeds (sunflower, sesame, pumpkin and flaxseed).

4. Combine the lime and flaxseed oil in a small bowl. Now, pour the mixture over the vegetables.

Dinner

Cheese and Zucchini Quiche (Serves 12)

Fat and protein ingredients:

12 large organic eggs or 15 medium eggs

5 cups of Colby jack cheese

Other ingredients:

2 cups of thinly sliced fresh zucchini+ 1 medium onion sliced thin

1 ½ cups of heavy cream+ 3 tablespoons of olive oil

2 teaspoons of oregano

1 ½ teaspoon of black pepper powder

Directions:

1. Preheat the oven to 350F.

2. Take 2 deep 10-inch quiche pans. Grease them with a bit of olive oil and keep aside.

3. Take a large mixing bowl. Crack all the eggs and pour into the bowl. Then add the heavy cream, oregano, pepper powder and beat well until it has all been mixed well.

4. Take each quiche pan and place the zucchini and onion slices evenly in each pan. Then sprinkle the cheese over them and finally pour the egg and cream mixture over it.

5. Bake for 20 minutes until the top is golden brown in color. Prick with a fork until bottom of quiche to check if done.

Day 3

Breakfast

Bacon & olive omelet (Serves 4)

Fat and protein ingredients:

8 large eggs

16 thin slices bacon

Other ingredients:

20 pitted black olives

Pinch of pink Himalayan or sea salt

Black pepper, freshly ground

Directions:

1. Cut the olives into thin slices.

2. Lay the bacon, preferably free-range or organic, equally on the surface of the pan and roast for about 5 minutes.

3. Break the eggs open into a large mixing bowl with a pinch of salt and pepper and whisk well with a wooden spoon, or fork.

4. Turn the bacon on the other side when it gets slightly golden in color.

5. Lower the heat and pour the egg mixture equally all over the pan. Don't rush it and don't try to cook it fast or it will end up being too crispy and dry.

6. Use a spatula to bring in the omelet from the sides towards the center for the first 30 seconds.

7. Sprinkle with sliced olives and cook for another minute or until the top appears to be almost cooked and firm.

8. Using a knife or a spatula, smooth out the edges of the omelet, remove the eggs from the heat and the pan from the heat, and serve it hot on a plate.

Lunch

Mixed Greens Salad (Serves 4)

Fat and protein ingredients:

4 tablespoons of grated Parmesan

4 slices Bacon

6 tablespoon of pine Nuts, roasted

Other ingredients:

4 oz. Mixed Greens

2 tablespoon apple cider vinegar

4 packets cooking Splenda or Stevia

Salt and Pepper to taste

Directions:

1. Place greens in a salad bowl

2. In a small bowl, mix the vinegar and stevia to create sweet/sour vinegar dressing.

3. Fry the bacon strips in its own fat until crisp. Crumble the bacon or cut in tiny strips.

4. Add the bacon, cheese, nuts, and dressing to the greens and toss until fully mixed.

Dinner

Creamed Brussels Sprouts (Serves 4)

Fat and protein ingredients:

5 tablespoons butter, divided

½ cup heavy cream

2 tablespoons grated Parmesan cheese

½ cup crushed pork rinds

Other ingredients:

2 cloves garlic, minced

2 cups sliced Brussels sprouts

½ teaspoon salt

1/2 teaspoon black pepper

Directions:

1. Preheat oven to 350°F.

2. Heat 2 tablespoons butter in a medium skillet over medium-high heat. Add garlic and sauté for 3 minutes.

3. Add Brussels sprouts and continue to sauté until Brussels sprouts

are fork tender, about 5 minutes.

3. Transfer Brussels sprouts, garlic, and melted butter to a 9" × 9" baking dish.

4. Add cream, Parmesan cheese, salt, and pepper.

5. Sprinkle pork rinds evenly over the top of Brussels sprouts and top with remaining butter.

6. Cover and bake for 30 minutes. Serve hot.

Day 4

Breakfast

Fresh Keto Style Egg Breakfast (Serves 2)

Fat and protein ingredients:

6 organic eggs

½ cup of heavy cream

1 tablespoon of butter

Other ingredients:

1 cup of shredded spinach

A small pinch of sea salt+ ground white pepper

1 small onion finely minced

Directions

1. Take a mixing bowl. Add the eggs, cream, salt and pepper and beat well and keep aside.

2. Take a large skillet and heat 1 tablespoon of butter.

3. Then add the onion and spinach and stir constantly.

4. Next, pour the egg mixture and stir until everything becomes scrambled and cooked till light, fluffy and yellow.

5. Serve hot.

Lunch

Spinach Salad (Serves 4)

Protein and fat ingredients:

3-4 tablespoons blue cheese. crumbled

1/2 cup bacon, cooked and crumbled

1/4 cup slivered macadamia nuts or slivered almonds, chopped

Other ingredients:

1/2 cup red onion, thinly sliced

3 to 4 cups washed baby spinach leaves

Directions:

1. In four plates, evenly place the spinach leaves.

2. On the spinach leaves, place the red onions evenly.

3. Sprinkle the nuts, cheese, bacon, and the spinach.

4. Use some store-bought low carb dressings, and spoon these over the spinach.

Dinner

Sea Bass with Mango Chutney, Ginger, and Black Sesame Seeds (Makes 2 servings)

Fat and protein ingredients:

Two 6-ounce striped bass fillets

1 tablespoon sesame oil

Other ingredients:

Cooking spray

1 tablespoon minced fresh ginger (see note)

1 tablespoon soy sauce

Salt and freshly milled black pepper to taste

¼ cup mango chutney

3 cups shredded iceberg lettuce

Ginger and Hot Red Pepper Vinaigrette

Directions:

1. Preheat the oven to 425°F. Spray an 8 X 8 X 8-inch Pyrex baking dish with cooking spray.

2. Place the fillets in the baking dish. Sprinkle each fillet with ginger, soy sauce, and sesame oil. Lightly salt and pepper. Cover the dish with foil and bake for 10 minutes.

3. Remove from the oven and spoon 2 tablespoons of chutney onto each fillet. Return to the oven and bake, uncovered, for 5 more minutes.

4. Toss the shredded lettuce with the dressing. Divide between two plates and top each one with a fillet.

Day 5

Breakfast

<u>Breakfast Muffins</u>

Fat and protein ingredients:

1 medium Egg

1/4 cup Heavy Cream

1 slice cooked Bacon (Cured, Pan-Fried, Cooked)

1 oz. Cheddar Cheese

Other ingredients:

Salt & black pepper (to taste)

Directions:

1. Preheat oven to 350 F

2. In a bowl, whisk the eggs with the cream and salt and pepper.

3. Spread into pam sprayed muffin tins, and fill the cups 1/2 full.

4. Place 1 slice crumbled bacon to each muffin and then 1/2 oz. cheese on top of each muffin.

5. Bake for about 15-20 minutes or until slightly browned.

6. Add another 1/2 oz. of cheese onto each muffin and broil until cheese is slightly

browned. Enjoy!

Lunch

Chicken Kebabs (Serves up to 5)

Protein and fat Ingredients:

10 6" rosemary skewers (soaked in water for at least 1 hour)

1.5lbs chicken tenderloins (approx. 10)

1/2 tablespoon rosemary olive oil (or regular)

Other ingredients:

A few sprigs of fresh thyme

1/2 tablespoon garlic salt

1/2 tablespoon lemon pepper seasoning

Instructions:

1. Preheat oven to 350 degrees Fahrenheit.

2. Soak the rosemary skewers for at least 1 hour in water

3. Use a short sharp knife to whittle a point on the end of each of each stick.

4. Toss chicken with ingredients. Slide the leaves off the thyme sprigs and sprinkle them in.

5. Skewer each piece of tenderloin with a rosemary stick.

6. Bake at 350 for 40 minutes

Dinner

Broccoli and Ham Quiche (Serves 12)

Fat and protein ingredients:

10 large organic eggs or 12 medium eggs

2 cups of thinly sliced ham

1 cup of grated cheddar cheese

44

1 ½ cups of heavy cream

3 tablespoons of olive oil

Other ingredients:

12 cups of cubed broccoli flowerets

2 teaspoons of chili flakes

Directions:

1. Preheat the oven to 350F.

2. Take 2 deep 10-inch quiche pans. Grease them with a bit of olive oil and keep aside.

3. Take a large mixing bowl. Crack all the eggs and pour into the bow. Then add the heavy cream, chili flakes, and beat well until it has all been mixed well.

4. Take each quiche pan and place the ham slices and broccoli flowerets evenly in each pan. Then sprinkle the cheese over them and finally pour the egg and cream mixture over it.

5. Bake for 20 minutes until the top is golden brown in color. Prick with a fork till bottom of quiche to check if done. If it is clean, then the quiche is ready to enjoy.

Day 6

Breakfast

Eggs Benedict (Serves 4)

Fat and other ingredients:

8 large eggs

2 tablespoon butter

8 slices sugar-free Canadian bacon

2 cups Hollandaise Sauce

Other Ingredients:

1 large avocado, cut into 8 pieces

Directions:

1. Heat up a medium skillet over medium-high heat and add the butter. Crack eggs into the pan. Cook for 2 minutes and then flip eggs, using care not to break yolks.

2. Cook for another 2 minutes or until white is completely cooked, but yolk is still runny.

3. Transfer eggs to a plate.

4. Top each egg with a slice of Canadian bacon and a slice of avocado. Pour some of the Hollandaise sauce onto each egg.

Lunch

Prawn Salad (makes 2 servings)

Fat and protein ingredients:

7 oz. king prawns, cooked

3.5 ounces smoked wild salmon

2 tablespoon virgin olive oil

Other ingredients:

2 cups cherry tomatoes

3 cups lettuce

2 teaspoon Dijon mustard

2 teaspoon wine vinegar

Two ounces' fresh ground black pepper

2 tablespoons contemporary dill

Instructions:

1. Begin by washing and draining the lettuce. Consider using a salad spinner.

2. Unfold the leaves evenly in a salad bowl.

3. Wash and halve the cherry tomatoes and add them to the bowl.

4. Slice the smoked salmon into skinny stripes and add them to the salad.

5. Add the prawns to the salad.

6. Make the dressing by mixing further virgin olive oil, crimson wine vinegar and Dijon mustard.

Dinner

Baked Salmon (Serves 4)

Fat and protein ingredients:

4 6-ounce salmon fillets

3 tablespoons olive oil

Other ingredients:

2 tablespoons of lemon juice

1 tablespoon each of minced parsley, mint, garlic, paprika, sunflower seeds (slightly crushed)

Directions:

1. Clean the fillet and put aside.

2. Place all the other ingredients in another bowl, and mix well and pour on the fish. Marinate the fillet for 6 hours.

3. After 6 hours, place in a baking dish and bake for 1 hour at 250F until flaky and cooked.

4. Serve with sour cream, green beans, and apricots.

Day 7

Breakfast

Pumpkin Pancakes (Serves 12)

Fat and protein ingredients:

1 ½ cups of cream cheese

3 eggs

¼ cup of melted butter

Other ingredients:

1 cup of steamed and pureed pumpkin

1 cup of coconut flour

½ teaspoon of chili flakes

1/3 teaspoon of pumpkin spice

2 teaspoons Stevia

Directions:

1. Take a large bowl and add the pumpkin, cream cheese, coconut flour, eggs, pumpkin spice, stevia, chili flakes and melted butter and mix well.

2. Keep aside covered for 15 minutes.

3. Take a non-stick pan and heat it. Once hot, pour a ladle of the pancake mixture and reduce the heat. Wait for 2 minutes and then flip over. Once golden and fluffy, place it onto a plate.

4. Serve hot with a dab of butter

Lunch

Chicken Salad (Serves 4)

Salad Ingredients:

Fat and protein ingredients:

2 cups cooked chicken, diced

Other ingredients:

1/2 cup sliced green onion

1/2 cup diced celery

Dressing ingredients:

Fat and protein ingredients:

3 ounces' mayonnaise

3 ounces' cream cheese, softened

Other ingredients:

1/2 teaspoon dried thyme

1 teaspoon dried tarragon

Salt and pepper to taste

Directions:

1. In a large bowl, mix the mayonnaise and cream cheese, and whisk the mixture until it achieves and smooth consistency.

2. Whisk in the thyme and tarragon.

3. Combine the chicken and vegetables and mix in with the dressing, making sure that the ingredients are coated. The salad may also be rolled up in the lettuce leaves lettuce leaves, and eat like a wrap.

Dinner

Fried Chicken (Serves 4)

Fat and protein ingredients:

1 pound or 4 (4-ounce) boneless, skinless chicken breasts

1/2 cup crushed pork rinds

1/2 cup grated Parmesan cheese

2 large eggs

2 tablespoons coconut oil

Other ingredients:

1/2 teaspoon garlic powder

1/4 teaspoon onion powder

1/4 teaspoon dried minced onion

1/4 teaspoon salt

1/4 teaspoon black pepper

Directions:

1. Put pork rinds, Parmesan cheese, garlic powder, onion powder, minced onion, salt, and black pepper in a large mixing bowl and stir until well mixed.

2. Crack eggs into a separate bowl and whisk.

3. Dip each chicken breast into eggs and then coat in pork rind mixture, making sure the chicken is completely covered.

4. Heat coconut oil in a skillet over medium-high heat. When coconut oil is hot, place chicken breasts into pan. Let cook for 5–7 minutes or until pork rind crust is browned. Flip chicken over and let cook for another 5–7 minutes until cooked through.

5. Serve hot.

Day 8

Breakfast

<u>Easy Spanish Omelets (Serves 2)</u>

Fat and protein ingredients:

3 eggs

Other ingredients:

Cayenne or black pepper

½ cup finely chopped vegetables e.g. olives, onions, chives, capsicum, parsley,

Spinach, zucchini.

Directions:

1. In a medium pan lightly stir-fry vegetables in extra virgin olive oil and remove

2. Cook eggs with one tablespoon of water and pinch of pepper.

3. When almost cooked top with vegetables and flip to heat through.

Lunch

Quick Cobb Keto Salad (Serves: 2)

Fat and protein ingredients:

2 large boiled hen eggs cut into small pieces

4 slices of fried bacon chopped coarsely

6 sausages diced and sautéed in1 tablespoon of olive oil

4 tablespoons of mayonnaise

4 tablespoons of heavy cream

2 tablespoons of olive oil

Other ingredients

1 cup of diced cucumbers

½ cup of boiled snap peas

¼ cup of pine nuts

1 teaspoon of mustard paste

1 tablespoon of vinegar

1 tablespoon of dill and mint leaves each

A dash of pepper

Directions:

1. Take a small bowl and add the mustard paste, mayonnaise, heavy cream, olive oil, vinegar, dill, mint leaves and pepper and mix well and keep aside. The dressing is ready.

2. In a large bowl, add the cut eggs, bacon bits, dices sausages, snap peas, and cucumbers, and pine nuts and finally pour in the dressing.

3. Mix well and serve warm or cold.

Dinner

Grilled Halibut with Anchovy-Lemon Butter (Serves 2)

Fat and protein ingredients:

Two 6-ounce halibut steaks

½ teaspoon extra-virgin olive oil

2 teaspoons softened unsalted butter

Other ingredients:

½ teaspoon kosher salt

½ teaspoon cracked pepper

1 tablespoon anchovy paste or 1 tablespoon chopped canned anchovy

Zest of 1 lemon plus 1 tablespoon fresh lemon juice

Directions:

1. Preheat a large skillet, and then film it with oil. Meanwhile, pat the fish steaks dry, then salt and pepper them.

2. Brush each side with a little oil then place in the skillet and cook about 4 minutes per side.

3. Mix together the butter, anchovy paste, zest, and lemon juice in a small bowl.

4. Transfer the steaks to warmed dinner plates and top with a dollop of anchovy butter.

Day 9

Breakfast

Creamy scrambled eggs (Serves 1)

Fat and protein ingredients:

3 large free-range eggs

2 tablespoon Crème fraîche

1 tablespoon ghee or butter, grass-fed (or coconut oil)

Other ingredients:

Pinch of pink Himalayan or sea salt

Freshly ground black pepper

Optional ingredients (makes 1 serving)

2 large bacon slices

Directions:

1. Crack the eggs into a mixing bowl with a pinch of salt and pepper and beat them well with a whisk or fork.

2. Pour the eggs into a pan, add butter (or ghee) and turn the heat on.

3. Keep on low heat, while stirring constantly. Do not stop stirring as the eggs may get dry and loose the creamy texture.

4 Take off the heat, spoon crème fraîche in and mix well with the eggs. This will help the eggs cool down and stop cooking while keeping the creamy texture.

5. Place on a serving plate and try with crispy bacon slices.

Lunch

Cabbage and Bleu Cheese Salad (Serves 2)

Fat and protein ingredients:

1 cup crumbled blue cheese

4 tablespoon entire walnuts

4 tablespoon walnut oil

Other ingredients:

4 cups shredded pink cabbage

3 small apples

2 tablespoon wine vinegar

Himalayan or sea salt

Freshly floor black pepper

2 apricots

Instructions:

1. Wash the cabbage, inexperienced apple, apricot (if included) and drain

2. Grate the cabbage thinly utilizing a hand grater or meals processor.

3. Grate the apple utilizing medium dimension holes on a hand grater and add to the bowl with cabbage.

Optional: Cut the apricot into small slices.

4. Roughly crumble the blue cheese by hand.

5. For the dressing, Mix together the walnut oil, wine vinegar, salt and pepper in a bowl.

Dinner

Spiced Lamb Chops on a Bed of Mushrooms and Spinach (Serves 2)

Fat and protein ingredients:

4 lamb rib chops, frenched

1 tablespoon olive oil

Other ingredients:

1 teaspoon coriander seeds

1 teaspoon ground cumin

2 teaspoons sweet paprika

½ teaspoon salt

1 tablespoon garlic powder

1 tablespoon water

Instructions:

1. Mix together the coriander, cumin, paprika, salt, garlic powder, olive oil, and water to make a paste in a small bowl.

2. Rub the spice paste on the lamb chops and let marinate for about 10 minutes.

3. Preheat a dry skillet over medium-high heat. Film with oil and add the chops. 4. Sauté for medium-rare about 3 minutes, or longer for desired level of doneness. 5. Arrange

half of the Mushroom and Spinach mixture on each of two plates.

6. Arrange the chops on top with the rib bones crossed.

Day 10

Breakfast

<u>Bacon Hash (Serves 4)</u>

Fat and protein ingredients:

6 slices sugar-free bacon

Other Ingredients:

2 cups chopped cauliflower

1 medium onion, diced

2 cloves garlic, minced

½ teaspoon salt

½ teaspoon black pepper

½ teaspoon garlic powder

Directions:

1. Fry the bacon in its own fat, in a medium skillet over medium heat until crispy. This could take up to 10 minutes.

2. Remove this from the pan and let cool, and then dice.

3. Add the chopped cauliflower, diced onion, and minced garlic to the skillet. Cook this for 5 minutes over medium heat, or until cauliflower starts to brown. Add salt, black pepper, garlic powder, and diced bacon. Stir until combined.

4. Remove from heat and serve.

5. This can actually be turned into a complete meal by adding a couple of poached or over-easy eggs on top. This versatile mixture can also be incorporated into scrambled eggs.

Lunch

Avocado and Cilantro Salad (Serves 4)

Fat and protein ingredients:

2 tablespoons avocado oil or extra-virgin olive oil

1/2 cup crumbled feta cheese

Other ingredients:

4 medium avocados, diced

1/2 cup chopped cilantro

2 tablespoons lemon juice

½ small white onion, sliced thinly

½ teaspoon salt

½ teaspoon black pepper

½ cup sliced pickled jalapeño peppers (optional)

Directions:

Combine all ingredients in a bowl and toss to coat.

Dinner

Pan-Grilled Pork Chops with Mango Glaze (Serves 2)

Fat and protein ingredients:

Two 5- to 6-ounce pork loin chops

Other ingredients:

1 teaspoon whole black peppercorns

½ cup vinegar (preferably white wine)

¼ teaspoon sugar

Half of a medium mango, diced and peeled

¼ teaspoon freshly milled black pepper

Salt to taste

Directions:

1. Transfer the vinegar to a small saucepan and boil over a medium-high heat. Add the sugar, diced mango, and peppercorns.

2. Keep cooking until the mixture is thick syrup, with the volume reduced by about a third. This will take from 4 to 5 minutes. Put this mixture aside.

2. Place a heavy iron skillet over medium to high heat. With some paper towels, dry the chops by gently patting them with paper towels. Add salt and pepper to taste.

3. Grill in the pan for about 5 minutes per side to get medium doneness.

4. Serve hot with a couple of spoonful of mango glaze atop each.

Day 11

Breakfast

Basic Steak and Eggs (Serves 4)

 Fat and protein ingredients:

Four4 oz. sirloin steaks

4 tablespoon butter

12 eggs

Other ingredients:

1 avocado

Salt and pepper to taste

Directions:

1. Melt the butter in a frying pan and cook the eggs until the yolk is done to your liking, and the whites are set. Season the eggs with pepper and salt, to taste.

2. In another pan, sauté the steak until done to your liking.

Slice or cube the steak according to your liking and dash with salt and pepper.

3. Add sliced avocado and serve.

Lunch

Deli Roll-Ups (Serves 2)

Fat and protein ingredients:

8 ounces' sugar-free deli ham, sliced

1/2 cup chive cream cheese

Other ingredients:

1 cup chopped baby spinach

1 red bell pepper, sliced

Directions:

1. Lay out each slice of ham flat.

2. Take 1 tablespoon of cream cheese and spread it on a slice of ham. Repeat for the remaining slices.

3. Put 2 tablespoons of chopped spinach on top of the cream cheese on each slice.

4. Divide bell pepper into 8 equal portions and put each portion on top of spinach.

5. Roll up the ham and secure with a toothpick. Eat immediately or refrigerate until ready to serve.

Dinner

Garlic Lime Chicken (Serves 2)

Fat and protein ingredients:

2 boneless, skinless chicken breasts (10 ounces total), split and pounded to ¼-inch thickness

Other ingredients:

2 tablespoons low sodium soy sauce

Grated zest and juice of 1 lime

1 teaspoon Worcestershire sauce

1 garlic clove, minced

½ teaspoon dry mustard

½ teaspoon cracked black pepper

Directions:

1. Combine the soy sauce, lime juice and zest, Worcestershire sauce, garlic, and mustard in a glass dish or resalable plastic bag.

2. Add the chicken and turn to coat with the mixture. Cover the chicken and refrigerate for 20 minutes.

3. Remove the chicken from the marinade and pepper it thoroughly. Discard the marinade.

4. Preheat a grill or skillet over medium-high heat. Film it with olive oil. Cook the chicken until golden on both sides and opaque and cooked through, about 10 minutes in total.

5. Serve hot or at room temperature garnished with additional lime zest.

Day 12

Breakfast

Breakfast Sausage Casserole (Serves 4)

Fat and protein ingredients:

8 eggs, beaten

1 lb. sausage, cooked and crumbled

2 cups heavy whipping cream

1 cup sharp cheddar cheese, grated

Other ingredients:

1 head of chopped cauliflower

1 teaspoon salt

1 teaspoon dry mustard

Directions:

1. Cook the sausage

2. In a medium bowl add together sausage, heavy whipping cream, chopped cauliflower, cheese, eggs, salt and mustard and mix well.

3. Pour into a 9×13 casserole dish that has been sprayed with Non-stick spray.

4. Cook for 45 minutes at 350 degrees F or until firm

5. Remove and top with more cheese

Lunch

<u>Sausage Balls (Serves 10 – good to store)</u>

Fat and protein ingredients:

2 cups of sausages shredded

½ cup of cheddar cheese

½ cup of cottage cheese

1 egg

1 tablespoon butter

Other ingredients:

1 teaspoon of chili flakes

½ cup of red peppers

¼ teaspoon of mustard powder

Directions:

1. Preheat an oven to 350 degrees.

2. Add the egg, chili, red peppers in a bowl and whisk until the ingredients are mixed completely.

3. Mix in the remaining ingredients.

4. Using a wooden baking spoon, or cookie scoop, remove the mixture, and hand-roll the sausage into about two dozen sausage balls.

5. Place the formed balls on a buttered baking pan, or cookie sheet

6. Bake for about 15 minutes. Serve.

7. You may also store the cooked sausage bags in a covered bowl, or sandwich bags in the refrigerator for later use.

Dinner

Rosemary Beef Medallions with Red Pepper Sauce (Serves 2)

Fat and protein ingredients:

10 ounces' beef tenderloin cut into ½-inch-thick rounds

1 teaspoon olive oil

2 tablespoons butter

Other ingredients:

¼ cup fresh lime juice

1 teaspoon dried rosemary, crushed

¼ cup roasted red bell peppers, drained well and chopped

Pinch of cayenne, to taste

Salt to taste

Directions:

1. In the bowl of a food processor with the blade removed, melt the butter in the microwave on high (full power) for 30 seconds.

2. Remove from the microwave, replace the metal blade in the food processor bowl and add the lime juice, rosemary, roasted red pepper, cayenne, and salt.

3. Pulse the mixture until thoroughly mixed. Taste and adjust the seasoning and set aside.

4. Heat a large dry skillet. Film with the oil, add the beef medallions, and sauté until golden, for 5 minutes per side for medium-rare.

5. Spoon the sauce onto two plates; arrange the meat in the pools of sauce.

Day 13

Breakfast

Egg-Chicharonnes Tortilla (Serves 2)

Protein and fat ingredients:

5 large eggs

4 slices Bacon

1.5 oz. Pork Rinds

Other ingredients:

1 medium Avocado

1 medium Tomato

1/4 cup Cilantro, chopped

2 medium Jalapeno Peppers, de-seeded

1/4 medium Onion

Salt and Pepper to Taste

Directions:

1. Dice the tomato, jalapeno peppers, and onion in preparation for cooking the other ingredients.

2. Fry the bacon. When done, place these on paper towels and set aside. Do not discard the bacon fat left in the pan.

3. Fry the pork rinds in the pan with the bacon fat until crispy, ensuring that the rinds are properly coated.

4. Add the vegetables to the pork rinds in the pan, and season as mix, as needed.

5. When the onions are almost "cooked", add the cilantro and mix well.

6. Scramble the eggs and add this to the mixture in the pan, seasoning as needed.

7. Cook the mixture as if it is an omelet, mixing the uncooked eggs to the bottom of the pan.

8. Cube the avocado immediately prior to serving and fold this into the egg dish.

Lunch

Pork Tacos (Serves 4)

Fat and pork ingredients:

25 oz. pork mince

½ cup of goat cheese

½ cup of mayonnaise

Other ingredients:

3 teaspoons Taco Seasoning

4 Romaine Lettuce Leaves

Directions:

1. Place the pork mince in a skillet and cook it for 20 minutes until nice and brown. Leave to cool.

2. Place the pork mince on the lettuce leaves.

3. Add the seasoning, goat cheese, and a dollop of mayonnaise.

4. Wrap securely.

Dinner

<u>Baked Zucchini (Serves 4)</u>

Fat and protein ingredients:

2 tablespoons extra-virgin olive oil

1 -1/2 cups shredded mozzarella cheese

½ cup full-fat ricotta cheese

2 tablespoons cream cheese

Other ingredients:

¼ cup chopped yellow onion

4 medium zucchini, julienned

1-1⁄2 cups Marinara Sauce or flavored tomato sauce

2 cloves garlic, minced

¼ cup chopped fresh basil

¼ cup chopped fresh oregano

½ teaspoon salt

½ teaspoon black pepper

Directions:

1. Preheat oven to 350°F.

2. Heat olive oil in a large skillet over medium heat and add onion. Sauté until translucent which could take about 3 minutes or less, and then add zucchini. Sauté for another 4 minutes or until zucchini is softened, but still firm.

3. Add / cup mozzarella cheese, ricotta cheese, cream cheese, marinara, garlic, basil, oregano, salt, and pepper to the pan. Bring to a simmer and remove from heat once cream cheese is melted.

4. Transfer to an 8" × 8" baking dish. Top with remaining mozzarella and bake for 15 minutes or until cheese is melted and casserole is bubbling.

Day 14

Breakfast

Egg Salad Breakfast (Serves 4)

Fat and protein ingredients:

12 large eggs

2 tablespoons of butter, melted

1/2 cup mayonnaise

Other ingredients:

1 teaspoon black pepper

1/2 teaspoon ground mustard

1 teaspoon salt

1/3 cup finely minced white onion

Directions:

1. Lay in eggs in a large pot filled with cold water.

2. Boil the eggs for 10 minutes.

2. Remove the pot from the heat, and then pour out as much hot water out as possible. Refill the pot with cold water, leaving the eggs in.

3. Leave the eggs to sit in the pot from 2-3 minutes.

4. Remove the eggs, patting them dry. Peel the eggs.

5. Cut the eggs into even 1/4 inch pieces. If you have an egg slicer, all the better.

6. Mix in the remaining ingredients thoroughly, and refrigerate until this is ready to serve.

Lunch

Stuffed Avocados (Serves 4)

Fat and protein ingredients:

2 (6-ounce) cans tuna in oil

4 tablespoons mayonnaise

Other ingredients:

2 large avocados

1 medium green bell pepper, chopped

1 teaspoon dried minced onion

1 teaspoon garlic salt

1 teaspoon black pepper

Directions:

1. Cut avocado in half lengthwise and remove the pit. Set aside.

2. Put tuna, mayonnaise, bell pepper, dried onion, garlic salt, and black pepper in a medium mixing bowl and mash together with a fork until combined.

3. Scoop half of the mixture into each half of the avocado.

Dinner

Roasted Butterfish (Serves 4)

Fat and protein ingredients:

Four giant butterfish fillets

8 tablespoon butter or ghee

Other ingredients:

4 cloves garlic

4 teaspoons freshly chopped thyme

Pinch sea salt

Juice from 1 lemon

Directions:

1. Begin by seasoning the recent (or defrosted) butterfish fillets with a little bit of salt to style and place them on a plate.

2. Soften the butter, add the herbs and crushed garlic and blend all the pieces collectively in a small bowl.

3. Pour the butter combination over the fish.

4. Warm a non-stick pan over medium heat and add the fish.

5. Roast for about 2-three minutes on both sides till cooked by and the fish will get a crispy golden texture. Be certain that the fillet is totally cooked by slicing into it. Cooked flesh will look opaque.

6. Place the fish onto a serving plate and squeeze a little bit of lemon over it. Serve sizzling.

Day 15

Breakfast

Ham, Cheese, and Egg Casserole (Serves 6)

Fat and protein ingredients:

12 large eggs

2 cups cooked diced sugar-free ham

1/2 cup shredded mozzarella cheese

1/2 cup shredded Cheddar cheese

Other Ingredients:

4 cups broccoli florets

1/2 cup chopped scallions

Bunches of broccoli (approximately one cup)

Directions:

1. Preheat oven to 375°F.

2. Fill a large pot with water and bring to a boil. Blanch broccoli by putting in boiling water for 2–3 minutes.

3. Put eggs, ham, mozzarella, cheddar, and scallions in a large bowl and whisk until combined. Add broccoli.

4. Pour into a 9" × 13" baking pan

Lunch

Tuna Steaks with Tarragon Mayonnaise (Serves 2)

Fat and protein ingredients:

Two 6-ounce tuna steaks, 1 inch thick

2 teaspoons mayonnaise

1 teaspoon olive oil

Other ingredients:

2 tablespoons minced fresh or 2 teaspoons dried tarragon plus tarragon sprigs for garnish

Salt and cracked pepper to taste

Directions:

1. Stir the mayo and tarragon together in a small bowl. Cover and set aside.

2. Heat a heavy skillet or ridged grill pan over medium-high heat.

3. Pat the tuna dry with paper towels, then season to taste with salt and cracked pepper. Dab olive oil over the surfaces of the fish.

4. Pan grill the fish about 3 minutes per side for medium. Transfer to warmed dinner plates.

5. Top each steak with a dollop of tarragon mayonnaise, and garnish with tarragon sprigs. Place a mound of squash beside the tuna.

Dinner

Broccoli Beef Stir Fry (Serves: 4)

Fat and protein ingredients

One pound of ground beef

5 tablespoons of coconut oil

1 cup of coconut milk

Other ingredients:

2 cups of chopped red onions

2 tablespoons of minced garlic

1/ 2 tablespoon of minced ginger

2 cups of chopped broccoli

½ cup of chopped fennel

1 cup of yellow peppers

1 cup of chopped mushrooms

1 teaspoon of cayenne pepper

Salt

Directions:

1. Heat a large wok and pour the coconut oil into it.

2. Throw in the garlic and red onions and stir. Then add the ground beef and stir. Cover and let it get cooked for 20 minutes.

3. Open the lid and add the fennel, yellow peppers, mushrooms, cayenne pepper, salt and stir for 5 minutes.

4. Pour in the coconut milk and add the broccoli, stir, and cover and cook for 5 minutes.

5. Open and check whether the stir fry is dry and ground beef has become well browned.

Day 16

Breakfast

Breakfast Keto Hash (Serves 4)

Fat and protein ingredients:

8 slices bacon

4 tablespoons ghee or coconut oil

Other ingredients:

4 tablespoons freshly chopped parsley or chives

2 teaspoons salt

4 large eggs free-range or organic on top

2 avocados

4 medium zucchini

2 cloves garlic

Directions:

1. Finely chop the garlic, and cut the bacon.

2. Cook the onion over medium heat and add the bacon, cook until lightly browned.

3. Meanwhile, dice the zucchini into medium pieces.

4. Add the zucchini to the pan and cook for 10-15 minutes.

5. Remove and add chopped parsley.

Lunch

Organic Chicken Salad (Serves 4)

Fat and protein ingredients:

Four 3 to 4 oz. chicken breast pieces

4 slices of bacon cut into small bits

Other ingredients:

1 tablespoon of peri peri sauce mix

1 cup of arugula leaves

½ cup of diced avocado

Juice of one lemon

Directions:

1. Heat a large frying pan and fry the bacon bits.

2. Then add the chicken breasts and fry until golden brown.

3. Take a bowl and add the arugula leaves, peri peri sauce, diced avocado, and the chicken and bacon bits.

4. Finally add the lemon juice and toss well and serve.

Dinner

Sriracha Bacon-Wrapped Shrimp (Serves 4)

Fat and protein ingredients:

1-pound medium sized frozen shrimp

8 strips bacon

Other ingredients:

¼ cup sriracha sauce

Directions:

1. Line a baking sheet with aluminum foil

2. Preheat the oven to 400 degrees.

3. Thaw frozen precooked medium sized shrimp and dry with a paper towel.

4. Cut bacon strips into two.

5. Spoon sriracha over the shrimp.

6. Wrap each shrimp with bacon, and secure with a toothpick.

7. Bake for about 20 minutes or until your bacon reaches the desired crispiness.

Day 17

Breakfast

Cheese and Onion Quiche (Serves 4 to 6)

Fat and protein ingredients:

12 large eggs

5-6 cups Colby jack or Muenster cheese, shredded

2 cups heavy cream

Other ingredients:

1 large onion, chopped finely

1 teaspoon ground black pepper

1 teaspoon salt

2 teaspoons dried thyme

Directions:

1. Set the oven to 350 degrees.

2. In a large skillet, melt the butter in medium-low heat.

3. Sauté the vegetables until the onions are soft and translucent. Remove the vegetables, and set aside.

4. Coat two deep pie pans or two 10-inch quiche pans with butter. Add two cups of shredded cheese in each pan.

5. Mix in 1/2 of the cooled cooked vegetable mix to each of the pans evenly over the cheese.

6. Break open the eggs and pour these into a large mixing bowl. Mix in the spices and cream, and then whisk until frothy.

7. Pour 1/2 of the mixture into each pan of the vegetables and cheese, and using a fork, distribute the cheese and vegetables evenly into the cream and egg mixture.

5. Place quiche pans into the oven, careful to leave about an inch between the pans. Bake for 20 minutes or so, or until slightly golden brown in the center, and puffy.

6. Slice the quiche into 6 evenly sized servings (total of twelve servings). This can be served immediately, or can be kept in a freezer for up to weeks, or refrigerated for a week.

Lunch

Warm Wild Mushroom and Chicken Salad in Balsamic Vinaigrette (Serves 2)

Fat and protein ingredients:

2 boneless, skinless chicken breasts (10 ounces total), split and pounded to ¼-inch thickness

2 tablespoons extra-virgin olive oil

½ teaspoon sesame oil

Other ingredients:

1 tablespoon balsamic vinegar

½ teaspoon dried thyme

2 tablespoons finely chopped fresh chives

Salt and freshly milled black pepper to taste

8 ounces assorted wild mushrooms

2 shallots, finely chopped

2 cups mesclun or mixed baby greens

Directions:

1. Stir together 2 tablespoons of the olive oil, the vinegar, thyme, and 1 tablespoon of the chives in a medium bowl. Set aside.

2. Toss the chicken breasts with 1 tablespoon of the olive oil and the salt and pepper.

3. Heat a dry medium skillet over medium-high heat for 2 minutes.

4. Add 2 tablespoons of the olive oil and sauté the chicken for 5 to 7 minutes per side, until well done.

5. Add to the bowl of dressing and hold.

6. Toss the mushrooms in the sesame oil and sauté with the shallots for 3 minutes. Cover and continue to cook for 5 to 7 minutes, stirring occasionally, until the mushrooms are tender.

7. Toss the cooked mushrooms and shallots with the chicken and vinaigrette. 8. Remove the chicken pieces and mushrooms from the dressing and toss in the mesclun greens. Toss thoroughly and divide the greens between two dinner plates, top with the chicken, and then the mushrooms.

8. Garnish with the remaining chives.

Dinner

Bacon & Onion Casserole (Serves 4)

Fat and protein ingredients:

1 cup diced sausage

6 pieces' bacon

5 eggs

1 tablespoon heavy whipping cream

1 cup shredded cheddar cheese

Other ingredients:

Quarter cup chopped onion

Salt/pepper to taste

Directions:

1. Preheat oven to 400.

2. Lay bacon on foil covered sheet pan and bake for 12-15 mins; set aside to drain on paper towel.

3. Reduce oven heat to 350.

4. Chop onions and put on the baking sheet in the bacon grease. Broil onions on high for about 5 minutes.

5. Chop sausage and add to a greased baking dish.

6. Mix eggs and cream together until completely combined.

7. Add the salt and pepper to your liking. Poor egg mixture over sausage and then add in your onions.

8. Cover with half of the cheese and then top with all your crumbled (or chopped) bacon.

9. Top with remaining cheese.

10. Bake on 350 for 30 minutes. Let cool for 5 minutes before serving.

11. Top and serve with a dollop of sour cream or mayonnaise.

Day 18

Breakfast

Quick Morning Scramble (Serves 4)

Fat and protein ingredients:

12 eggs, whisked

8 slices of deli ham

4 tablespoon of coconut oil or ghee

1 tablespoon butter

Other ingredients:

16 baby bella mushrooms

1/2 cup red bell peppers

1 cup of spinach

Salt and pepper to taste

Directions:

1. Chop up the vegetables and the ham.

2. Place butter into a frying pan and melt. Sauté the vegetables and ham.

3. Place the whisked eggs into a separate frying pan with the other ½ tablespoon of butter. Cook on medium heat and keep stirring to prevent overcooking.

4. Once the eggs are cooked, season them with salt and pepper to taste.

5. Add the sautéed vegetables and ham in with the eggs and mix. Serve immediately

Lunch

Mushroom and Chicken Salad in a Balsamic Vinaigrette (Serves 2)

Fat and protein ingredients:

2 boneless, skinless chicken breasts (10 ounces total), split and pounded to ¼-inch thickness

2 tablespoons extra-virgin olive oil

½ teaspoon sesame oil

Other ingredients:

2 tablespoons finely chopped fresh chives

Salt and freshly milled black pepper to taste

8 ounces assorted wild mushrooms

2 shallots, finely chopped

2 cups mesclun or mixed baby greens

1 tablespoon balsamic vinegar

½ teaspoon dried thyme

Directions:

1. Stir together 2 tablespoons of the olive oil, the vinegar, thyme, and 1 tablespoon of the chives in a medium bowl. Set aside.

2. Toss the chicken breasts with 1 tablespoon of the olive oil and the salt and pepper.

3. Heat a dry medium skillet over medium-high heat for 2 minutes. Add 2 tablespoons of the olive oil and sauté the chicken for 5 to 7 minutes per side, until well done. Add to the bowl of dressing and hold.

4. Toss the mushrooms in the sesame oil and sauté with the shallots for 3 minutes. Cover and continue to cook for 5 to 7 minutes, stirring occasionally, until the mushrooms are tender.

5. Toss the cooked mushrooms and shallots with the chicken and vinaigrette.

6. Remove the chicken pieces and mushrooms from the dressing and toss in the mesclun greens. Toss thoroughly and divide the greens between two dinner plates, top with the chicken, and then the mushrooms.

7. Garnish with the remaining chives.

Dinner

Meatball "Sub" (Serves 6, making 18 meatballs)

Fat and protein ingredients:

1-pound ground beef

12/pound ground pork

2 tablespoons grated Parmesan cheese

6 slices provolone cheese

2 large eggs

Other ingredients:

¼ cup chopped fresh basil

2 tablespoons minced fresh parsley

1 tablespoon minced garlic

1 teaspoon salt

¼ teaspoon black pepper

1 cup Marinara Sauce or flavored tomato paste

Directions:

1. Preheat oven to 325°F.

2. Mix beef, pork, Parmesan cheese, eggs, basil, parsley, garlic, salt, and pepper in a large mixing bowl until well combined.

3. Roll meat mixture into 1" balls and place about 1" apart on a baking sheet. Bake until cooked through, about 15 minutes. Remove meatballs from the oven and set aside to cool for a few minutes.

4. Place 1 slice of provolone cheese flat on a plate and put 3 meatballs on one side of it.

5. Pour the marinara sauce over the meatballs. Fold the other side of the cheese over the meatballs.

Day 19

Breakfast

Egg muffins with goat cheese (Serves 6)

Fat and protein ingredients:

4 large free-range eggs

1 1⁄2 cup frozen spinach

1 cup crumbled feta cheese

6 thin slices bacon

Other ingredients:

1⁄2 teaspoon pink Himalayan or sea salt

Directions:

1. Preheat the oven to 350°F/175°C. Use a microwave to defrost the spinach or leave overnight at room temperature.

2. Cut the bacon into small stripes and add them to a non-stick pan. Roast until slightly browned and remove from the heat.

3. Crack the eggs into a bowl and whisk them well. Season with salt (but don't put too much because feta cheese is quite salty as well).

4. Divide the spinach, feta and bacon evenly into the muffin forms and add crumbled feta. If you cannot eat dairy, use roasted mushrooms or more bacon.

5. Pour over with the eggs and transfer into the oven.

6. Bake for 20-25 minutes until golden brown. Enjoy hot or cold.

Lunch

Sesame-Crusted Chicken on a Bed of Bean Sprouts (Serves 2)

Fat and protein ingredients:

2 boneless, skinless chicken thighs (10 ounces total)

1 large egg white, lightly beaten

2 tablespoons peanut oil

Other ingredients:

½ teaspoon ground cinnamon

½ teaspoon white pepper

¼ teaspoon fennel seeds

¼ teaspoon kosher salt

1 garlic clove, crushed

Grated zest from ½ lemon plus 1 teaspoon fresh lemon juice

1 tablespoon all-purpose flour

1 tablespoon toasted sesame seeds

3 cups chilled bean sprouts

1 teaspoon low sodium soy sauce

1 teaspoon grated fresh ginger

Directions:

1. Place the thighs in a glass dish.

2. Mix the soy sauce, ginger, cinnamon, white pepper, fennel seeds, salt, and garlic in a small bowl.

3. Pour over the chicken. Cover and set aside for 10 to 15 minutes.

4. Meanwhile, in a medium bowl, whisk the egg white with the lemon zest and juice until foamy.

5. Sprinkle the chicken pieces with the flour, and then dredge in the egg mixture.

6. Preheat a large skillet over medium-high heat, and then add the oil.

7. Add the chicken and cook about 6 minutes on each side, or until cooked through.

8. Divide the bean sprouts between two dinner plates.

9. Top with cooked chicken and serve.

Dinner

Ginger Beef (Serves 2)

Fat and protein ingredients:

2 cups of thinly sliced beef strips

5 tablespoons of sesame oil

Other ingredients:

1 cup of cauliflower flowerets

1 cup of diced mushrooms

½ cup of string beans cut into 1 inch pieces

2 tablespoons of vinegar

2 tablespoon of soy sauce

2 tablespoons of tomato sauce

2 cups of diced onion

1 cup of red peppers

3 tablespoons of minced ginger

1 tablespoon of minced garlic

Directions:

1. Heat a large wok and pour 5 tablespoons of sesame oil. Put in the ginger and garlic and stir.

2. Add the onion, peppers, and the beef and stir for 5 minutes. Let it cook for 10 minutes, on medium heat and with lid on.

3. Take off the lid and add the mushrooms, cauliflowers, and beans. Keep on stirring while cooking on high heat for 5-8 minutes.

4. Add the vinegar, soy sauce and tomato sauce and stir and serve hot.

Day 20

Breakfast

Scrambled Eggs with Bacon (Serves 4)

Fat and protein ingredients:

8 slices bacon

12 large eggs

1/2 cup heavy cream

Other Ingredients:

1/2 teaspoon salt

1/2 teaspoon black pepper

Directions:

1. Cook bacon in a medium skillet over medium heat until crispy, about 10 minutes. Remove bacon from pan and dice.

2. Crack eggs into a medium bowl and whisk together with heavy cream, salt, and pepper. Add egg mixture to bacon grease in pan and stir until scrambled. Add diced bacon to eggs and stir.

3. Remove from heat and serve immediately.

Lunch

<u>Mahi-mahi with Roasted Red Peppers (Serves 2)</u>

Fat and protein ingredients:

12-ounce mahi-mahi fillets

1 ½ tablespoons extra-virgin olive oil

Other ingredients:

2 roasted red bell pepper, chopped

1 clove garlic, minced

¼ teaspoon cumin

1 tablespoon fresh lemon juice

½ teaspoon salt

½ teaspoon freshly milled black pepper

Directions:

1. Preheat the oven to 425°F.

2. Spray an 8 X 8 X 8-inch Pyrex baking dish with cooking spray or oil lightly.

3. Stir the red pepper, garlic, cumin, lemon juice, and 1 teaspoon of the olive oil into the dish.

4. Lay mahi-mahi fillets on top and brush with the remaining oil.

5. Season lightly with salt and pepper. Cover tightly with aluminum foil. Bake for 12 to 15 minutes, just until the fish is opaque.

6. Scoop red pepper and fish onto warmed dinner plate.

Dinner

Meatloaf (Serves 12)

Fat and protein ingredients:

2 cups of minced pork

2 cups of shredded sausage meat

10 slices of bacon chopped

½ cup of cheddar cheese

½ cup of parmesan cheese

4 eggs

5 tablespoons of cold milk

½ cup butter

Other ingredients:

¾ cup of almond flour

1 tablespoon gelatin

2 cups of chopped onions

1 cup of green peppers

8 cloves of garlic minced

2 basil leaves

2 all spice leaves

2 bunches of parsley leaves- all chopped finely

4 tablespoons of vinegar

2 tablespoons of honey

2 tablespoons of barbeque sauce

Salt and pepper to taste

Directions:

1. Take a large baking dish and grease it with butter. Keep aside.

2. Preheat oven to 350 degrees.

3. Take a frying pan, add butter, then add the onions, green peppers, and garlic and bacon and sauté for two minutes and keep aside.

4. Soak the gelatin in the cold milk and keep aside.

5. In a large mixing bowl, add pork mince, sausage meat, almond flour, cheddar cheese, parmesan cheese, eggs, soaked gelatin, sautéed onion mixture, the spice leaves, salt, pepper, vinegar, barbeque sauce, honey, and the rest of the butter and mix well.

6. Ensure that it becomes somewhat like non-sticky dough. You may add more almond flour and cheese until you get this consistency.

7. Place the mixture inside a baking dish and bake at 180 degrees for about one hour.

8. Insert a knife inside the loaf and if it comes out clean, then the meat loaf is cooked.

8. Cool for 20 minutes, then slice and serve it with sour cream and salad.

Day 21

Breakfast

One Skillet Bacon and Eggs (Serves 4)

Fat and protein ingredients:

8 slices bacon

4 large eggs

½ cup shredded Colby jack cheese

1 tablespoon butter

Other ingredients:

½ large white onion, chopped into small pieces

1 carrot, cut into thin strips

½ cup celery, finely chopped

½ cup chopped broccoli or cauliflower

Directions:

1. Cut up the bacon into smaller strips.

2. In a large pan or skillet, melt the butter over medium heat.

3, Add the bacon and vegetables.

4. Sauté the vegetables and bacon in the butter, stirring often. Cook them for about 15 minutes, or until the vegetables begin to caramelize, and the bacon strips begin to get crispy around the edges.

5. Mix the eggs into the mixture until the eggs are almost cooked.

6. Sprinkle the cheese over the eggs when the eggs are nearly done, and cook a little more, until the cheese is melted.

Lunch

Tomato Salad (Serves 2)

Fat and protein ingredients:

4 tablespoon virgin olive oil

Other ingredients:

1 cup cherry tomatoes

3 cups rocket (arugula)

1 small purple onion

4 tablespoon drained canned capers

2 tablespoon basil

Directions:

1. Wash the rocket and drain properly on a paper tissue or in a lettuce strainer. Place it on a serving plate or right into a serving bowl.

2. Wash, drain and halve the tomatoes. Add them into the bowl with the rocket.

3. Chop the onion and recent basil thinly and add to the bowl. Prime with capers and toss with olive oil.

Dinner

Halibut with Capers (Serves 2)

Fat and protein ingredients:

Two 6-ounce boneless, skinless halibut fillets

1 tablespoon butter

1 tablespoon peanut oil

Other ingredients:

½ teaspoon salt

½ teaspoon freshly milled black pepper

1 tablespoon all-purpose flour

½ cup low-sodium chicken broth

Grated zest and juice of 1 lemon

1 tablespoon drained capers

Directions:

1. Stir together the salt, pepper, and flour on a piece of wax paper.

2. Mix the broth, lemon, and capers in a small cup. Heat a large skillet over medium-high heat, and then film the bottom with oil.

3. Dredge the fish in the seasoned flour, and then cook until it is light brown on the bottom, about 2 minutes. Flip it over, adding oil if necessary to keep it from sticking, and cook the second side until browned, about 2 minutes.

4. Transfer to warmed dinner plates. Crank up the heat under the skillet and pour in the lemon-caper mixture.

5. Scrape up the brown bits in the skillet and boil it down until somewhat reduced. Remove from the heat, and swirl in the butter.

6. Pour the sauce over the fish and serve

Day 22

Breakfast

Cajun Cauliflower Mix (Serves 2)

Fat and protein ingredients:

8 oz. shaved red pastrami (chopped into 1" slices)

2 tablespoons olive oil

Other ingredients:

1-lb bag frozen cauliflower (steamed and then chopped into small even chunks)

1/2 onion (chopped into 1/4 inch pieces)

1/2 green pepper (chopped into 1/4 inch pieces)

2 tablespoons minced garlic

1 teaspoon store-bought Cajun seasoning

Directions:

1. Sauté' the chopped onions in the olive oil for about 5 minutes over medium heat.

2. Sauté the garlic for about2 minutes.

3. Squeeze remaining water from the cauliflower and mix it into the sauté for about 5-10 minutes until the cauliflower begins to turn crisp, and brown.

4. Mix in the Cajun seasoning.

5. Mixed in the green peppers and chopped pastrami.

6. Continue cooking for about 5 minutes, and serve hot.

Lunch

Roast Beef Lettuce Wraps (Serves 4)

Fat and protein ingredients:

8 ounces (8 slices) rare roast beef

1⁄2 cup mayonnaise

8 slices provolone cheese

Other ingredients:

8 large iceberg lettuce leaves

1 cup baby spinach

Iceberg Lettuce

Directions:

1. Wash lettuce leaves and pat them dry, being careful not to rip them.

2. Place 1 slice of roast beef in each lettuce wrap.

3. Spread / tablespoon of mayonnaise on each piece of roast beef.

4. Top mayonnaise with 1 slice of provolone cheese and / cup of baby spinach.

5. Roll lettuce up around toppings. Serve immediately.

Dinner

Lamb Chops with Blueberry Vinegar Reduction (Serves 2)

Fat and protein ingredients:

Two 6-ounce lamb loin chops

2 tablespoons olive oil

½ cup heavy cream

Other ingredients:

2 garlic cloves, finely chopped

½ small tomato, minced

¼ cup blueberry or other fruit vinegar

¾ cup low-sodium chicken broth

½ cup fresh blueberries

Salt and freshly milled black pepper to taste

Directions:

1. Heat the oil in a medium skillet over medium-high until almost smoking.

2. Add the lamb chops and brown for about 3 minutes on each side. Remove from the heat and hold on a warm plate.

3. Add the garlic to the pan and sauté for 30 seconds or until fragrant.

4. Add the tomato, vinegar, broth, and cream, and cook over medium heat until reduced by half, 3 to 5 minutes.

5. Return the chops to the pan with any of their juices and cook, uncovered, for 3 more minutes.

6. Add the blue-berries and cook for 1 more minute.

7. Taste and add salt and pepper to taste. Serve at once.

Day 23

Breakfast

Spiced Strawberries (Serves 4)

Ingredients:

2 cups halved strawberries

1 tablespoon sugar

2 teaspoon sherry vinegar

¼ teaspoon finely milled black pepper

Directions:

Toss the berries with the sugar, vinegar, and pepper in a medium bowl. Cover and chill for at least 15 minutes. Serve in footed dessert dishes.

Lunch

Ball Park Mustard Chicken on a Bed of Baby Spinach (Serves 2)

Fat and protein ingredients:

2 boneless, skinless chicken breasts (10 ounces total), split and pounded to ¼-inch thickness

¼ cup plain yogurt

1 teaspoon olive oil

Other ingredients:

1 tablespoon ball park (or other spicy) mustard

¼ teaspoon kosher salt

¼ teaspoon cayenne

One 12-ounce package baby spinach

Directions:

1. Preheat the oven to 400°F. Stir the yogurt, mustard, salt, and cayenne together in a bowl.

2. Rub the chicken breast cutlets with the yogurt mixture and place on a greased baking sheet. Roast about 20 minutes, or until cooked through.

3 In the meantime, wash the spinach leaves, but do not dry.

4. Heat a large skillet, and then film it with oil.

5. Add the spinach by the handful. Cook and stir until the spinach is limp.

6. Transfer to two warmed dinner plates. Top with chicken breasts and serve.

Dinner

Steamed Snapper with Blue Cheese Spread (Serves 2)

Fat and protein ingredients:

2 fillets of snapper

1 cup of blue cheese

¼ cup of heavy cream

Other ingredients:

2 tablespoons of lemon juice+ 2 cloves of garlic minced

Salt and pepper to taste

1 bunch of coriander leaves chopped finely

1 tablespoon of prawn crackers

Directions:

1. Take a steamer and place the fish on the top basket. Sprinkle salt, pepper, and lime juice over it and steam for 10 minutes.

2. Take a bowl, and place the blue cheese and heavy cream and salt and pepper and beat well until light. Then fold in coriander leaves and prawn crackers.

3. Serve the blue cheese spread with the steamed snapper and some vegetables of your choice.

Day 24

Breakfast

Keto Breakfast Burrito (Single serving)

Fat and protein ingredients:

Sliced Ham (make sure the pieces are big enough so that they can be used to fold up or roll-up, burrito style, or you may need to use more than a slice for each roll)

2 large eggs

1 teaspoon olive oil

Other ingredients:

1/4 cup chopped vegetables, such as black olives, tomatoes, bell peppers, or spinach

You can also use store-bought bottled salsa

Directions:

1. In a pan, sauté the vegetables over high heat in a small bit of oil over medium high heat.

2. Whisk the eggs in a medium heat, and pour the eggs over the veggie mix.

3. Scramble the mixture with a wooden spoon, or spatula until it is cooked through. Remove the eggs from the pan when cooked.

4. Wrap the ham around the egg mixture and return this into the skillet.

5. Cook this for 10-15 seconds, or until each side of the ham is slightly brown.

5. Serve with guacamole, salsa, and fresh cilantro.

Lunch

<u>Chopped Chicken Salad with Romaine (Serves 2)</u>

Fat and protein ingredients:

8 ounces roasted chicken breast, chopped into bite-size pieces

1 tablespoon coarsely chopped dry-roasted peanuts

Other ingredients:

¾ cup chopped red apple (Macintosh or other puckery sweet varieties)

¼ cup chopped celery

Dressing ingredients:

¼ cup plain yogurt

1 tablespoon mayonnaise

½ teaspoon curry powder

¼ teaspoon kosher salt

Pinch of cayenne

4 cups coarsely chopped romaine lettuce leaves

Directions:

1. Toss together the chicken, apple, celery, and peanuts in a large bowl.

2. In a small bowl, stir together the ingredients for the dressing.

3. Toss with the chicken mixture.

4. Arrange the lettuce leaves on two plates, mound the chicken mixture on top, and serve.

Dinner

Savory beef steaks (Serves 4)

Fat and protein ingredients:

4 medium venison steaks

8 tablespoon butter or ghee, grass-fed (or coconut oil)

Other ingredients:

6 tablespoon spiced cranberry relish (dwelling-made)

2 tablespoons balsamic vinegar

Pinch of pink Himalayan or sea salt

Directions:

1. Allow the steaks to sit down at room temperature for 10-quarter-hour. Use a paper towel to pat the surplus blood off. Toss with a few of the melted ghee (or butter, tallow, lard) and season with salt.

2. Fry in an extremely popular heavy based mostly pan greased with ghee over excessive warmth for two-three minutes on both sides to seal within

Day 25

Breakfast

<u>Baked Spinach and Mozzarella (Serves 4)</u>

Fat and protein ingredients:

8 large eggs

1 tablespoon olive oil

3/4 cup shredded mozzarella cheese

3/4 cup shredded Colby jack cheese

Other ingredients:

4 cups baby spinach

1/4 cup chopped scallions

1/2 teaspoon salt

1/2 teaspoon black pepper

Directions:

1. Preheat oven to 375°F.

2. Heat olive oil in a medium skillet over medium heat and add spinach. Sauté until wilted. Transfer spinach to a 9" × 9" baking dish.

3. Put remaining ingredients in a medium bowl and whisk until combined. Pour egg mixture on top of spinach.

4. Bake for 30 minutes or until eggs are no longer runny. Serve warm.

Lunch

Bacon Broccoli Salad (Serves 4)

Fat and protein ingredients:

1/2 lb. Bacon

1 cup Mayonnaise

1 teaspoon Sesame oil

Other ingredients:

2 lbs. Broccoli florets

1 1/2 oz. Green onion

2 tablespoon White vinegar

Directions:

1. Fry the bacon in its own fat.

2. When cooked, crumble the bacon into small pieces.

3. Combine the bacon with all the other ingredients in a salad bowl.

Dinner

<u>Bacon-Wrapped Asparagus (Serves 4)</u>

Fat and protein ingredients:

6 slices sugar-free bacon

Other ingredients:

12 asparagus spears, ends trimmed

Directions:

1. Cut each strip of bacon in half lengthwise.

2. Wrap a piece of bacon around each asparagus spear and secure in place with a toothpick.

3. Grill over medium heat for 10 minutes, or until bacon is crisp, turning each spear over halfway through cooking time.

Day 26

Breakfast

<u>Super Quick Scramble Recipe (Single serving)</u>

Fat and protein ingredients:

3 eggs, whisked

2 slices of deli ham

1 tablespoon of coconut oil or ghee

Other ingredients:

4 baby bella mushrooms

¼ cup red bell peppers

½ cup of spinach

Salt and pepper to taste

Directions:

1. Chop up the vegetables and the ham.

2. Place ½ tablespoon of butter into a frying pan and melt. Sauté the vegetables and ham.

3. Place the whisked eggs into a separate frying pan with the other ½ tablespoon of butter. Cook on medium heat and keep stirring to prevent overcooking.

4. Once the eggs are cooked, season them with salt and pepper to taste.

5. Mix in the sautéed vegetables and ham. Serve immediately.

Lunch

Waldorf Salad (Serves 4)

Protein and fat ingredients:

3 ounces full-fat cream cheese

2 tablespoons unsalted ghee or butter or ghee

1/2 cup blue cheese, crumbled

Other ingredients:

1/2 small green apple, diced into 1/2-inch pieces

1/4 teaspoon onion powder

1/4 teaspoon garlic powder

2 tablespoons spring onion and fresh chives, chopped

2/3 cup pecans or walnuts, roughly chopped

Pepper, to taste

Salt, to taste

Directions:

1. In a bowl, mix cream cheese with the ghee butter or ghee until smooth.

2. Mix in the chives, onion powder, apple and crumbled blue cheese, apple, garlic powder. Season with pepper and salt.

3. Place the refrigerator for about twenty minutes, or until set.

4. Using a large wooden spoon, convert the mixture into 6 evenly sized balls. Roll the cooked balls onto the pecans.

Dinner

Buttered Pork Kebabs (Serves 4)

Fat and pork ingredients:

16 cubes of pork meat (4 pieces per person)

¼ cup unsweetened butter

Other ingredients:

16 green pepper cubes

16 red onion cubes

8 pineapple cubes

2 tablespoons of garlic powder

1 tablespoon of brown sugar

2 tablespoons of soy sauce

1 teaspoon of chili flakes

½ teaspoon of almond flour

Directions:

1. Take a large bowl; add the pork cubes, peppers, onion and pineapple cubes, and the sunflower butter, garlic powder, brown sugar, soy sauce, chili flakes and mix well. Marinade for one hour or overnight.

2. Heat a grill pan and spray oil on it.

3. Now place each pork cubes on the grill and cook for 10- 12 minutes on each side. Keep aside when cooked.

4. Next place the onions, peppers and pineapple and grill for 2 minutes on each side. Keep aside when cooked.

5. Pour the marinade onto the grill pan. Let it boil then add the almond flour.

6. Stir quickly and also add the pork cubes, onions, peppers and pineapple cubes. Toss quickly to evenly coat the pieces with the glossy marinade.

7. Serve hot Kebabs with Lettuce leaves and apricots.

Day 27

Breakfast

Baked Bacon and Eggs (Serves 2)

Fat and protein ingredients:

8 slices cooked bacon, crumbled

4 large eggs

2 tablespoons butter

1 cup cheddar cheese, grated

1 cup heavy cream, lukewarm

Other ingredients:

Pepper and salt to taste

Directions:

1. Pre-heat an oven to 350 degrees. Coat four 6 oz. or so ramekins, with butter.

2. Break an egg into the individual ramekins.

3. Cover the eggs with 1/4 cup of cheese, 1/4 cup of heated cream, and, and add the pepper and salt.

4. Put the ramekins in a large pan and fill the pan with cold water. Place enough water so that the water will reach about half of the ramekins' height.

5. Place in the oven for about fifteen minutes, or until the egg whites are cooked fully or the cheese has been melted.

6. Sprinkle the crumbled pieces of two cooked bacon slices over the eggs of each ramekin, and serve hot.

Lunch

<u>Tuna and Egg Salad (Serves 2)</u>

Fat and protein ingredients:

2 large hard-boiled eggs

2 (6-ounce) cans tuna (try to get those packed in oil

1⁄2 cup mayonnaise

Other ingredients:

1⁄4 cup diced white onion

1⁄4 cup sugar-free relish

½ teaspoon salt

½ teaspoon black pepper

Directions:

1. Put eggs in a medium mixing bowl and mash with a fork. Add tuna and mayonnaise and mash together until ingredients are combined.

2. Stir in onion, relish, salt, and pepper.

Dinner

Mac n' Cheese (Serves 6)

Fat and protein ingredients:

3 ounces' cream cheese

1 cup heavy cream

1/cups shredded Cheddar cheese, divided

½ cup crushed pork rinds

Other ingredients:

6 cups cauliflower florets

1/2 teaspoon black pepper

1/2 teaspoon garlic powder

1/2 teaspoon salt

Directions:

1. Preheat oven to 375°F.

2. Fill a double boiler with water and bring water to a boil. Cut cauliflower into small pieces and place in the top portion of the double boiler. Steam until tender, which should take about 5 minutes.

3. Remove cauliflower from double boiler and place in a strainer.

4. Melt cream cheese in a medium saucepan over medium heat. Add heavy cream and whisk until combined. Whisk in 1 cup of Cheddar cheese, pepper, garlic powder, and salt. Once cheese has melted, remove from heat.

5. Transfer strained cauliflower to a 9" × 9" baking dish. Pour in cheese mixture and toss to coat cauliflower. Sprinkle remaining/cup of cheese and pork rinds on top.

6. Bake until bubbly, about 20 minutes.

Day 28

Breakfast

<u>Omelet with Goat Cheese and Herbs (Single serving)</u>

Fat and protein ingredients

3 large eggs

2 ounces' fresh goat cheese, crumbled

1 tablespoon unsalted butter

Other ingredients:

1/8 teaspoon Black pepper

½ teaspoon kosher salt

1 tablespoon herbs, such as basil, cilantro, or parsley, chopped

Directions:

1. Beat the eggs, and whisk together the eggs, salt, herbs, and the pepper.

2. In a small nonstick skillet, melt the tablespoon of butter

3. Mix in the eggs for about 3 minutes.

4. Sprinkle cheese over the eggs and fold the egg in equal halves. Cook for about one minute, or until the cheese is melted.

Lunch

<u>Chicken and Avocado Salad (Serves 2)</u>

Fat and protein ingredients:

1 (12.5-ounce) can shredded chicken breast

½ cup Homemade Mayonnaise

1 teaspoon olive oil

Other ingredients:

1 medium avocado, cubed

2 tablespoons sliced black olives

½ teaspoon garlic salt

½ teaspoon black pepper

¼ teaspoon paprika

1 teaspoon fresh lemon juice

Instructions:

Put all ingredients in a medium mixing bowl and mash with a fork until combined.

Dinner

Grilled Swordfish with Salsa (Serves 2)

Fat and protein ingredients:

Two 6-ounce boneless, skinless swordfish steaks, ¾ inch thick

1 tablespoon olive oil

Other ingredients:

2 cups shredded iceberg lettuce

1 cup sliced radishes

1 large avocado

2 tablespoons best-quality salsa pumped up with a little fresh cilantro

Grated zest and juice of 1 lime

Instructions:

1. Preheat the gas, charcoal, or electric grill.

2. Brush the fish with olive oil on both sides. Grill the fish, turning once after it has browned on the bottom (about 2 minutes), then finish on the second side, cooking until the fish is translucent in the middle (2 to 3 more minutes).

3. While grilling, make a bed of lettuce, radishes, and avocado on two warmed dinner plates.

4. Transfer the cooked fish to the dinner plates and top each steak with a big dollop of salsa.

5. Squeeze lime juice over the fish and sprinkle with zest.

Day 29

Breakfast

Skillet Soufflé (Serves 4)

Fat and protein ingredients

6 large eggs, with the yolks and egg whites separated

4 ounces' goat cheese

2 tablespoons extra-virgin olive oil

1 tablespoon unsalted butter

Other ingredients:

1 5-ounce store-bought bag salad greens

1/2 pint grape tomatoes, halved

1/4 cup chopped fresh chives

1 lemon, cut into wedges

1 teaspoon sea salt or kosher salt

1/4 teaspoon ground black pepper

Directions:

1. Preheat an oven to 400 F.

2. Mix together the egg yolks, pepper, salt, and chives, into a large bowl.

3. In another bowl, use an electric mixer, and with medium-high speed, beat the separated egg whites until stiff peaks appear. Gently fold the whites, using a spatula with the yolk mixture.

4. In a large nonstick skillet, melt the butter over medium heat and tilt the pan to coat the sides evenly.

5. Place egg mixture into the buttered skillet and sprinkle the crumbled cheese on top. Place the skillet in the oven, and cook until the eggs are golden and puffed. This will take about ten minutes.

6. Cut the cooked eggs into wedges. Divide the salad greens, tomatoes, and evenly between plates.

7. Drizzle the dish with the oil and lemon juice.

Lunch

Smoked Salmon Salad (Serves 2)

Fat and protein ingredients:

8 oz. smoked wild salmon

4 tablespoon mayonnaise

Other ingredients:

1 medium avocado

2 small spring onions

Juice from 1⁄2 lemon

Juice from 1⁄2 lime

1 teaspoon lime zest

Instructions:

1. Wash and chop the parsley and spring onion and place them in a salad bowl.

2. Peel the avocado, take away the seed and reduce it into skinny stripes. Squeeze some lemon over it to keep the avocado from turning brown.

3. Slice the smoked salmon and add it to the bowl with avocado.

4. Make the dressing by mixing mayonnaise with lime zest and lime juice.

5. Pour the dressing over the salad and revel in!

Dinner

Avocado-Lime Salmon (Serves 2)

Fat and protein ingredients:

2 6 oz. salmon fillets

Other ingredients:

1 avocado

1/2 lime

2 tablespoons red onion (diced)

100 grams' cauliflower

Instructions:

1. Place the cauliflower in a food processor until it resembles rice.

2. Remove the cauliflower from the processor, and cook that in a lightly oiled pan, covered, for about 10 minutes.

3. In a food processor, blend together an avocado, the lime juice, and diced red onion until smooth and creamy.

4. Heat a skillet with some oil and cook your salmon fillet skin side down for about 4-5 minutes. Season with salt and pepper while it's cooking.

5. Flip the salmon and continue to cook for an additional 4-5 minutes.

6. Once cooked, serve the fish over the bed of cauliflower rice, and a generous dollop of the avocado lime sauce.

Day 30

Breakfast

Steak and Eggs with Seared Tomatoes (Serves 4)

Fat and protein ingredients:

1-pound flank steak

4 large eggs

2 tablespoons olive oil (to be used in two even portions)

Other ingredients:

4 large tomatoes, halved

1 tablespoon fresh oregano, chopped

Kosher salt and black pepper

Directions:

1. Heat a tablespoon of olive oil in a large pan over medium heat.

2. Season the steak with ½ teaspoon pepper and ¼ teaspoon salt.

2. Grill the steak for about 5 minutes per side to get medium-rare doneness. Remove the steak from the skillet and set aside for five minutes before slicing.

3. Place the tomatoes to the skillet and cook, with the cut-side on the surface for about 2 minutes, or until browned.

4. Meanwhile, heat the remaining olive oil in a nonstick pan in medium heat.

5. Open the eggs into the skillet and cover, cooking to the desired doneness.

6. Sprinkle oregano, salt and pepper over the tomatoes, and serve with the steak.

Lunch

Spicy Chicken and Avocado Casserole (Serves 6)

Fat and protein ingredients:

3 (12.5-ounce) cans shredded chicken breast

1⁄2 cup sour cream

1⁄2 cup mayonnaise

1/2 cups shredded Cheddar cheese, divided

2 tablespoons coconut oil

Other ingredients:

2 large avocados, roughly chopped

1 small onion, diced

1 medium green bell pepper, diced

1/8 teaspoon red pepper flakes

1/4 teaspoon salt

1/4 teaspoon black pepper

Instructions:

1. Preheat oven to 350°F.

2. Spread chopped avocados along the bottom of a 9" × 13" baking pan.

3. Heat coconut oil in a medium skillet over medium-high heat. Add diced onions and cook until lightly browned, about 3 minutes. Add bell pepper to pan and cook until soft, another 3 minutes. Remove from heat.

4. Place chicken, sour cream, mayonnaise, 1 cup of Cheddar cheese, red pepper, salt, and black pepper in a medium mixing bowl and stir until combined.

5. Add onions and bell peppers.

6. Spoon mixture over avocados. Top with remaining/cup of Cheddar cheese.

7. Bake for 20 minutes or until cheese is slightly browned and casserole is bubbling.

8. Allow to cool slightly before serving

Dinner

<u>One Pan Baked Chicken Thighs (Serves 2)</u>

Fat and protein ingredients:

4 chicken thighs (deboned, skin on)

1/4 cup olive oil

Other ingredients:

2 zucchinis

1/2 cup carrot (sliced)

2 tablespoons balsamic vinegar

1 cup daikon radish

1-inch length of cube ginger, minced

Instructions:

1. Pre-heat an oven to 350 degrees.

2. Use a paper towel, and pat the chicken thighs dry.

3. Wrap the skins around the chicken thighs, and place these on a buttered or greased baking sheet.

4. Slice the radish and zucchinis, and with the carrots, place them around the thigh pieces.

5. To prepare the sauce, mix the vinegar, oil, and ginger in a bowl. Pour the mix over the chicken.

5. Season with salt and pepper and bake the chicken thighs for 30 minutes.

Atkins Diet

The Ultimate Guide to Atkins Diet

Table of Contents

Introduction

Weight loss is something that nearly everyone struggles with, especially as we get older. As our metabolism slows down, it is much easier to gain fat, lose muscle, and face new health ailments that keep us from enjoying life. If you do a simple google search about how to lose weight, thousands of articles, diet plans, and workout routines will immediately pop up. Of course, the general idea for any weight loss plan is to eat right and exercise, right? So, out of the hundreds of methods you can choose from, which one is right for you?

Atkins has been proven to be the most efficient and effective weight loss plan out there. It has helped millions of people around the globe find health and happiness through its strict but effective regiment. The question is, how do you know if Atkins will work for you and give you the results you want? The answer is simple. Atkins works for everyone whose goal is to burn fat and become healthier. This method in particular works because it keeps you from consuming foods that have any form of sugar, so that your body burns pure fat for energy instead.

The modern diet is largely made up of carbohydrates and fats, which do not work well together and contribute to the development of several diseases. This guide will teach you everything you need to know about the Atkins diet, as well as how your body functions using basic macronutrients. Through carefully laid out steps and strategies, you will learn how to become truly independent from sugar addiction, cravings, and common factors that attribute to falling off the wagon and going back to your old eating habits.

Here is an inescapable fact: most people will fail in their weight loss attempts. More than sixty- percent of the people who create goals and want to become healthier are unsuccessful and stay unhappy with their bodies. This guide gives you all the information you could possibly need to not only be successful in your journey of losing weight, but also become an inspiration and role model for other individuals who aspire to greater health. Knowledge is your greatest advantage to any new goal, and this book will teach you the science behind the Atkins diet, how cutting out carbohydrates can save your life, and a complete twenty – one-day meal plan to get you through the first phase of the program.

If you do not develop your understanding of weight loss, you will spend years looking for "the secret" or "magic supplement" that doesn't exist. Too many people look for the easiest way to get what they want, without acknowledging that the greatest success comes from a little struggle and a lot of willpower. Atkins is not just a dieting program, but the most trusted and effective strategy to burning fat and achieving your goals that you will ever find.

It's time for you to become an amazing and happier you. Think of all the things you will miss out on if you do not change your habits and lead a healthier life. Now is the time to take control of your lifestyle and change for the better. You *can* be skinner, toned, strong, and healthy; if you choose to be. It is time for you to begin your journey of transformation and rejuvenation. Good luck and enjoy!

Chapter 1: What is Atkins? The Game-Changing Weight Loss Plan

The theory of dieting has been around for as long as society has wanted a solution to their weight loss and health needs. There are dozens of cultures, religions, and countries around the world who all promote and live by different eating habits; all of which have their own benefits and disadvantages. The various lifestyles lead to the cultivation of hundreds of diet plans and programs that all promise to help you lose weight. An idea that was not often practiced in the twentieth century is now a multi- billion- dollar institution that promotes and feeds off of the public's insecurities and resolutions. However, it was not until recently that any of these methods were particularly effective.

We live in an age where food is accessible and cheap, which makes it easy to over eat and make poor choices with meals. Many diets share the same focus of cutting out calories, so that your body begins utilizing more calories than what you are intaking to create energy. This leads to less water weight and overall loss of fat, muscle, and water. The general foundation of this method works, but not to the fullest extent of what you truly want when changing your eating habits so drastically. Eating in a caloric deficit will allow you to lose weight, but it will not help you to keep the weight off for good. In fact, many diets often leave the participant hungry and craving sugar- loaded foods. After your body is starved of calories for so long, the individual experiences a great relapse and binges more than they have in the past. This leads to gaining back all of the weight that you just lost, and then some. The vicious cycle continues as another weight loss program is found and the individual picks up right where they initially began. Different diet, same concept.

The reality is that even though most diets are based off of cutting out calories, there is not much evidence that suggests doing so will manifest long- term success. Thus, the search for a diet that works on a different strategy for overall health and weight loss continues. This is where Atkins comes into play. What many have considered to be another fad diet, has brought success in the journey for long-term weight loss for anyone who has dared to take on the challenge of cutting out something other than calories from their diet. Atkins takes a more scientific approach to the theory of losing weight by analyzing how the modernized western diet has changed.

Today, we consume more carbohydrates than ever before and rely on bread and starch as staples for every meal. Cereal, pasta, and bread on consumed on a daily basis, which leads to the body storing more fat and living off the short bursts of energy that simple carbohydrates fuel. There is much to be said about how carbs and fats interact with your body's chemistry; however, that will be discussed in a later chapter.

The Atkins diet was made famous by physician Dr. Robert C. Atkins through is best- selling book that explained the diet in 1972. Since the release of his work, the Atkins diet has reached all four corners of the globe and inspired millions of people to look at weight loss with a different perspective. Many books and articles have reanalyzed and digested the diet time and time again, all with their own unique take on the matter. At first, the Atkins diet was deemed unhealthy and even confronted mainstream health authorities for their use of carbohydrates and saturated fat. However, there have been dozens of studies that have proven the many benefits that Atkins has to offer, despite what skeptics and critics may believe.

Atkins does not promote the idea of cutting out calories from your diet, but simple carbohydrates and sugar. This idea was entirely new, but proved successful for many. This is because when you reduce your carb intake and increase your protein intake, your appetite greatly subsides and end up consuming less calories without even realizing it. Diets that are high in carbohydrates leave your appetite satisfied for a short amount of time, as cravings and hunger pangs will ensue just an hour after eating. Atkins begins by completely cutting out carbs, and then slowly

170

reintroducing complex carbohydrates once your body has learned how to run efficiently without unnecessary sugar. There are several rules and guidelines that are outlined throughout the diet, however the complete long- term alteration of one's eating habits encourages individuals view Atkins as a lifestyle change, rather than a short- term solution to losing weight.

The key to staying successful with Atkins is sticking to it, even after the first phase is over. You will experience cravings and even perhaps lapses of judgement, just like you would have with any other dieting program. However, Atkins does not encourage you to keep to a restrictive regiment for too long, and reintroduces foods that you love as you learn how to correctly consume them in relation to the high consumption of protein and fat that Atkins requires. Now, you may be wondering how you could possibly give up bread and other sugary foods that have become staples to your diet. Once you have completed the first phase of the program, you will crave those foods less and be able to enjoy small amounts later on as you progress through the program.

Atkins Phases Broken Down

Phase 1:

Phase one is designed to help your body detox from sugar and become reliant on protein and fat for energy instead of carbohydrates. During this stage, you will consume under twenty grams of carbohydrates each day for approximately two weeks. Throughout the extent of phase one, you will eat meals that are high in fat, protein, and count your carbs through vegetables, like leafy greens.

Phase one allows your metabolism to kick- start into weight loss mode. So, that you can reprogram the way your body utilizes macronutrients. This first part of the programs is often mistaken for the structure of the entire program, but this is an inaccurate judgement. While you function off just twenty carbs a day, you begin understand the maximum grams of net carbs that you can

171

eat while also experiencing weight loss and adequate energy levels. This is referred to as your personal carb balance, which will be established as you continue into the next phase.

This phase should last for a minimum of two weeks, although you can safely follow the guidelines of this phase for as long as you need to if your goal is to lose as much weight as possible in the shortest amount of time. In this case, you will continue with phase one until you are fifteen pounds away from your target weight.

Phase 2:

Once you have achieved your goal weight with phase one, it is time to begin phase two. During this part of the diet plan, the participant will slowly start to add in new types of carbohydrates. The purpose is to correctly reintroduce the right kind of carbohydrates into your meal plan, so that you are still giving your body the nutrients it needs while still losing weight. You will begin eating nuts, low- carb veggies, and small amounts of fruit; and you will continue this phase until you are within ten pounds of your target weight.

Keep in mind that just because you can start eating carbs again does not mean that you can eat whatever you want, as long as it isn't too much. Nuts, strawberries, melon, seeds, cottage cheese, blueberries, and cottage cheese are a few examples of what you are limited to during phase two. The purpose of adding some more carbohydrates to your meal in this phase is to help you keep your momentum that you gained in the beginning of phase one, while still attempting to find your personal carbohydrate balance. Although you may stay dedicated to phase two until you are within ten pounds of your target weight, you can transition into phase three sooner if you are willing to let your weight loss pace slow a little.

Phase 3:

Phase three marks the progress that you have made, as you are closer than ever to your target weight. At this point in the Atkins plan, you will add even more carbohydrates into your diet until your weight loss slightly slows down. This phase is meant to help you fine- tune your diet so that you can eventually focus on maintaining your weight loss when you come into phase four. During phase three, you will see how much you can increase your daily net carb consumption while still maintaining weight loss during while reintroducing a wider variety of carbohydrate- filled foods. You will remain in phase three until you have achieved your goal weight and maintained it for at least thirty days.

Phase 4:

Phase four is designed to help you maintain your weight loss and new health diet. During this part of the Atkins plan, you are allowed to consume as many health carbohydrates as your body can take without paying close attention to your weight. This phase is regarded as a lifetime lifestyle, when you generally stick with the meal plan as a long- term commitment; eating the same foods that you have already been consuming with each new phase. Some foods that you may have tried to reintroduce earlier on, your body can now adequately handle. As long as you maintain your target weight, you can continue experimenting with small amounts of different carbs and other foods that you enjoy.

The phases that mark the progression of the Atkin diet may seem a bit complicated or even unnecessary. However, the entire program is designed to help your body overcome the addiction to carbohydrates while still enjoying the tasty foods that you love. The truth of the matter is that you are the only one who fully understands how your body works. You will notice right away if part of the meal plan does not work for you and your needs, and can easily alter your strategy accordingly. While giving up carbohydrates for any length of time can prove to be challenging, the first phase only lasts for two weeks and the benefits of detoxing from sugar can last a lifetime.

Chapter 2: The Basics of Atkins

Efficient protein intake and working your body into a ketogenic state are critical components to maximizing fat loss and maintaining muscle during the Atkins diet. While the first phase of Atkins may require a minimum of two weeks of dedication, it will take approximately three weeks for your body to become adapted to its natural ketogenic function. During the beginning phase of Atkins, nitrogen loss may occur if your carb consumption is extremely low. This is due to the fact that when your carb intake decreases, your body resorts to converting protein into glucose. Approximately sixteen percent of protein is nitrogen, and thus the loss of muscle occurs and your metabolic rate will decrease. Issues like this arise when you are not consuming adequate amounts of protein. Although your body is used to converting carbohydrates into glucose for energy, it can efficiently do this with protein and fats as well. The reason that our bodies do not already default to this way of functioning is because the modern diet is largely made up of carbohydrates and sugary foods; which are easier to break down into glucose.

This issue is especially inconvenient for body builders and other gym goers, as building muscle is essential for their regiment. So, how many carbohydrates do you need in order to maintain muscle and spare protein loss? The greatest challenge that comes with limiting your carb intake is that your body can go into starvation mode for too long, which leads to muscle loss. Starvation mode occurs when you consume less than fifteen carbs per day; this is necessary for your body to utilize its fat stores for energy. When you increase your carb consumption to fifty grams per day, your body is less dependent on amino acids for glycogenesis. Glycogenesis occurs through two different mechanisms. Firstly, when the increased carb consumption results in high blood glucose and insulin levels, which restricts your cortisol release. And secondly, when the carbs supply the brain with glucose, inhibiting the breakdown of protein in the body.

While keeping to the Atkins diet, your overall protein intake should account for at least seventy – percent of your diet; with your fat intake making up twenty – percent, and carbohydrates accounting for the remaining ten percent. As you move into the second phase, your carb intake will increase by ten percent, as your fat and protein intake decrease slightly. As you continue through the program, you will slowly alter the percentage of your macronutrient intake as your body adjusts to the new meal plan.

You can easily figure out how many grams of protein, fat, and carbohydrates you should consume with each meal and on a daily basis by using online macronutrient calculators. The website will ask a variety of questions based on your goals and physical health in order to determine the correct macro proportions for your diet. You will have to fill in information regarding your:

- Age

- Weight

- Sex

- Height

- Daily or Weekly Activity Level

    o Sedentary

    o Lightly Active

    o Moderately Active

    o Very Active

- The Kind of Exercise You Typically Perform

- Current Body Fat Percentage

- Main Objective Regarding Your Diet

    o Lose Weight

- o Maintain Weight
- o Gain Muscle

What to Eat on the Atkins Diet?

<u>Meat</u>

- Bacon
- Beef
- Fish/ Seafood
- Poultry
- Pork
- Turkey

<u>Eggs</u>

<u>Vegetables</u>

- Artichokes
- Asparagus
- Broccoli
- Cabbage
- Celery
- Cauliflower
- Kale
- Lettuce
- Mushroom
- Onions

- Peppers

- Radishes

- Spinach

- Spaghetti Squash

- Zucchini

Fats/Oils

- Coconut

- Flaxseed

- Olive

- Sesame

- Sunflower

Dairy

- Butter

- Cheese

- Full Fat Cream Cheese

- Full Fat Yogurt

- Heavy Whipping Cream

- Sour Cream

Nuts and Seeds

(All nuts are permitted during Phases 2-4)

Seeds:

- Chia

- Flax

- Pumpkin
- Sesame
- Sunflower

<u>Drinks</u>

- Water
- Tea (Black)
- Coffee (Black)

Foods to Avoid While on the Atkins Diet

<u>Breads and Grains</u>

- Bagels
- Barley
- Couscous
- English Muffins
- Kaiser Rolls
- Oats
- Pasta
- Rice
- Tortillas
- Products Containing Flour
- Whole Grains

<u>Vegetables</u> (During Phase One Only)

- Beans
- Carrots
- Chickpeas

- Corn
- Hummus
- Lentils
- Peas
- Potatoes
- Soy Beans
- Tomatoes
- Turnips

Sweets

- Cake
- Cookies
- Ice Cream
- Pastries
- Pies
- Pudding
- Gelatin

Sugars and Sweeteners

- White Sugar
- Brown Sugar
- Sucralose
- Aspartame
- Erythritol
- Agave Nectar
- Xylitol

Drinks

- Alcohol
- Energy Drinks
- Hot Chocolate
- Juice
- Milk
- Protein Shakes
- Soft Drinks
- Sports Drinks
- Sweetened Teas

Vegetable Oils and Fats
- Canola Oil
- Vegetable Oil
- Soybean Oil
- Trans Fats

High – Carb Fruits
- Apples
- Bananas
- Grapes
- Oranges
- Pears

Adding Carbs Back into Your Diet After Phase One

Despite what many people may believe, the Atkins program is relatively flexible. The most difficult part of beginning this diet is the first phase, in which you will minimize your carb intake. Once the induction phase is over, you are allowed to slowly integrate healthy carbohydrates back into your diet. This includes vegetables that are higher in carbohydrates, fruits, starches, and healthy grains such as oats and brown rice. However, once you have made it to the final phase of the program, you will need to maintain that lifestyle for the long haul; even if you have achieved your weight loss and health goals.

It is crucial that you keep to the diet you have formed during the final phase because your body will react differently to the old foods that you used to eat. You may have bloating and trouble digesting as your body becomes sensitive to certain foods that may be difficult for it to process. Regardless, even if your body does not have a negative reaction to high carbohydrate food products, you will gain back the weight you lose during the last three phases. Of course, this rings true for any weight loss program you try.

Atkins allows you to eat the delicious foods you love, such as bacon and cheese. However, as you begin introducing new foods during the second phase, you can experiment with different types of carbohydrates. As your net carb intake increases to fifty grams, you can start eating dark chocolate, fruits, oats, etc. One of the most difficult factors for many people on this diet is finding foods to snack on. While you may not be able to go to your default bag of potato chips or candy, there are plenty of options to keep you satisfied with your salty and sweet cravings. Some examples of low – carb snacks include:

- Hard – boiled eggs
- Cheese
- Nuts and seeds
- Yogurt
- Berries and whipped cream
- Green tea

Chapter 3: The Science Behind the Diet: Why it Works

We have been lead to believe that the more carbs and less fat we have in our diets, the healthier we will be. After all, carbohydrates are a source of energy, while fat makes us fat. Right? Actually, this way of thinking is completely wrong. Our bodies are capable of many things, and one of them is converting fat and protein into energy. Why would you want to completely change your diet just so your body uses fat for energy? Because fat does not make you fat: sugar does. In fact, carbohydrates are made up of starch, fiber, and sugar. When broken down during the digestive process, the majority of these nutrients are stored away for later as fat. This means that the more carbohydrates you eat, the more your body will store away for later, as it only takes a small number of carbs to function on a day to day basis.

Fat, on the other hand, does not get stored away as fat cells when you consume too much of it; and neither does protein. When you cut out carbs from your diet and increase the amount of protein and fat you eat, the way your body functions entirely changes. Its traditional energy source is no longer available, so it must resort to using other nutrients for energy. When this happens, your body begins using your stored fat as fuel, and you begin to lose weight. This process is called ketosis.

Ketosis is something that your body does every day, whether you eat carbs or not. However, eating a low carb, high fat diet gives this process a natural boost. Your body breaks carbohydrates down into glucose, because glucose is needed to create energy. When your body does not have glucose to process, it goes into a deep state of ketosis. Your body will burn fat stores, creating molecules: ketones. Ketones occur when your body breaks down fat into fatty acids in the liver during a process known as beta- oxidation. Although during the first few weeks of ketosis, the individual will experience energy lulls, studies have shown that your body runs up to seventy percent more efficiently than when it uses glucose for energy. This coincides perfectly with our evolution as human beings. Our ancestors did not have access to the food that we eat today, and therefore relied on protein and fat to keep them nourished.

While your body is in ketosis, it is possible that it produces too many ketone bodies. Therefore, the body with naturally expel of excess ketones through urine. However, this is not a sign that your state of ketosis is slowing down, but that your brains has enough BHB (beta- hydroxybutyric acid) to keep functioning at a higher level. Although the idea of burning pure fat sounds great, your body does need glucose to maintain maximum health, which is why phase one is the only time during Atkins when you will severely limit your carb intake.

Your body can theoretically completely become independent from carbohydrates. This is due to the breakdown of excess protein in your diet. Protein can be used for energy, building muscle, and keeping your bones strong. However, when you eat too much protein, approximately fifty- six percent will be turned into glucose in the bloodstream. Therefore, it is crucial that you keep a strict eye on your protein intake during the first three phases; so you don't accidently knock your body out of ketosis.

It is important to recognize that ketosis and starvation are two entirely different things. Starvation occurs when your body has no source of food or nutrition. This will result in muscle loss as your body begins using its own stores of protein in your muscles to stay alive. Ketosis is a temporary state of fasting that will encourage your body to use some of your fat stores for energy to induce weight loss. When done correctly, the ketogenic process will preserve your muscle tissue.

What to Expect During Phase One: Introducing Your Body to Ketosis

When you start any diet, you will notice weight loss almost immediately. However, this "weight loss" is not stored fat, but simply water weight. The human body is mostly made up of water. When you consume a lot of carbohydrates, you may experience bloating, even the day after consuming a big meal. This is because carbohydrate molecules and water molecules cling to each other, resulting in excess water weight. During the beginning of the Atkins diet, you will first drop any bloating that is caused by retaining water.

Once your body has dropped its water weight, you will start to lose real pounds of fat. Although it is easy to get hung up on the scale, it is more important to note the more obvious physical changes. While you may only drop a few pounds when you weigh in, your waist may have shrunk by a few inches. Lost inches are relatively more significant than numbers on a scale. Your clothes will feel a bit looser even if the number on the scale does not budge. During the Atkins program, is it normal for your body to fluctuate on a daily basis. Keeping a constant eye on the scale is not an efficient way of measuring your progress on this diet.

Carbohydrate- filled foods often contain massive amounts of sodium, which is not necessarily a bad thing. As your body flushes out toxins, ketones, and other excess nutrients, it will begin to lose electrolytes as well. If you begin feeling ill or a lack of energy, try drinking full sodium broth every day. This technique will also stop constipation, headaches, and muscle cramps during the first phase.

The best way to begin the Atkins program is to lose any expectations you may have. Everyone's body is different, and will react in different ways to the sudden change in diet. Your friend may have lost seven pounds within the first week of phase one, but there is no way of knowing if you will lose the same amount. Just know that during induction, you are cleansing your body in the most efficient way, and becoming a better and healthier you with each passing day.

Chapter 4: Top Benefits of Cutting and Limiting Carbohydrates

Low carb- high fat diets have been used for thousands of years for its various healing benefits. Nearly every culture in the world recognizes some form of this program as a way to cure diseases, improve overall health, and enhance the body's natural functions. While weight loss may be your primary reason for switching to a ketogenic diet, there are other benefits that you should consider while making this transition.

1. Inhibiting Your Appetite (In a Positive Way)

Hunger is not only eventually leads to bingeing, but it is also possibly the worst side effect of dieting. Hunger is typically the main reason most people feel terrible while dieting and end up giving up on losing weight all together. Let's face it, no one likes hunger pangs. Possibly the best part about switching to a low- carb diet is the automatic reduction of your appetite. Various studies have shown that when cutting down carbs and increasing protein and fat intake, people end up eating much fewer calories than normal. Without even trying, you will already eat less than usual.

2. More Weight Loss Than You Expect

It is no secret that cutting out carbohydrates is the simplest and by far most effective method of losing weight. After learning the biological process of burning fat on the Atkins diet, it is easy to see that people on low- carb diets tend to lose more weight quicker than individuals who stick to a low- fat meal plan. Even when others may restrict calories, people who adopt a ketogenic diet will still have more success.

This is due, firstly, to the quick explement of excess water weight from the body. Additionally, due to lower insulin levels, your kidneys will also get rid of extra sodium through urination, resulting in even more weight loss. When comparing studies, experts have found that individuals who keep to a low carb diet will lose up to three times as much weight, without experiencing hunger.

The most successful weight loss stories featuring low- carb diets report sticking to the diet for longer than six months. This is because many people tend to resort back to their old eating habits after reaching their goal weight. This is why sticking with a low – carb diet as your lifestyle will create better results, as long- term commitment soon becomes second nature.

3. Most of the Fat Loss Achieved in from the Abdominal Cavity

Even though we all would love to lose fat from everywhere on our bodies, the reality is that not all fat in your body is the same. Where your fat is stored dictates how your health is affected and whether or not you are at risk for disease. Your body contains two kinds of fat: subcutaneous and visceral. Subcutaneous fat is the layer underneath your skin, while visceral fat resides in your abdominal cavity and around your organs. Too much visceral fat results in increased inflammation, insulin resistance, and metabolic dysfunction disorder; commonly found in Westernized countries.

Low- carb lifestyles are extremely effective at decreasing excess fat around your abdomen, so that stubborn belly fat is more likely to disappear during the first few phases of Atkins. The reduction of visceral fat will also reduce your potential of developing heart disease and type 2 diabetes.

4. Your Triglyceride Levels Will Drastically Decrease

Triglycerides are fat molecules. An excess of triglycerides is when there is high level of fat is in your blood stream. Elevated triglyceride levels may result in the hardening of your arteries or the development of pancreatitis. It will also dramatically increase your risk of heart attack, heart disease, and stroke. It has become common knowledge in the medical world that fasting triglycerides (how much of them are in your blood after fasting overnight) is a strong indication of potential heart disease.

While many people believe that eating a lot of fat will result in elevated triglycerides, it is really carbohydrates that are the culprit; especially in the form of simple sugar. Cutting carbs results in the dramatic decrease of blood triglycerides, which is the exact opposite result of low- fat diets.

5. Improved Levels of HDL Cholesterol

Not many people know that cholesterol comes in two forms: LDL and HDL. HDL, high density lipoprotein, is known as the "good" cholesterol. LDL and HDL direct the lipoproteins that transport cholesterol through the bloodstream. LDL actually transports the cholesterol from the liver to the rest of your body, but HDL carries it away from the rest of the body towards the liver to be reused or disposed of. The more elevated your HDL cholesterol levels are, your risk of heart disease is drastically lowered. The most efficient method of improving your HDL cholesterol levels is eating a low-carb, high- fat diet. HDL levels may only increase moderately or even go down when consuming a low- fat diet.

6. Decreased Blood Sugar Levels and Insulin Levels: In Relation to Individuals with Type 2 Diabetes

Type 2 diabetes is somewhat of an epidemic this day and age: the rising child obesity rates and poor eating habits of adults has resulted in an increase of this condition throughout the population. When we consume carbohydrates, the molecules are broken down into simple sugars, like glucose), within the digestive tract. Once broken down, the glucose enters the bloodstream and results in elevated blood sugar levels. However, high blood sugar levels are extremely toxic. Therefore, your body responds by producing the hormone insulin. Insulin communicates to your cells that there is too much glucose and they need to bring it down by either burning it or storing it.

Individuals who are health have a quick insulin response, which minimizes the blood sugar spike to prevent too much glucose from harming our bodies. However, millions of people suffer from major problems with responding to glucose spikes. Those with type 2 diabetes suffer from insulin resistance; when their cells do not recognize the insulin and therefore have a more difficult time lowering the blood sugar levels using your cells. It is crucial that your body produces enough insulin after meals to quickly lower your blood sugar; so patients with type 2 diabetes will inject even more insulin into their bodies after eating.

Cutting out carbohydrates improve your body's response to glucose spikes by eliminating the need for so much insulin. Therefore, both blood sugars and insulin dramatically decrease. In fact, keeping to a strict low/ no- carb diet will cure type 2 diabetes altogether within just a few months. However, if you are taking blood sugar- lowering medication, you should consult your doctor before making changes to your diet in order to prevent hypoglycemia (dangerously low blood sugar.

7. Your Blood Pressure Will Go Way Down

Hypertension, or elevated blood pressure, is not only a symptom of many diseases, but also a risk factor for developing new conditions. Such ailments include heart disease, heart attack, stroke, thyroid issues, diabetes, kidney disease, kidney failure, and many other diseases. Low carb diets are one of the most effective methods of quickly reducing blood pressure, which will help decrease the risk of disease and help you live a long and happy life.

8. Extremely Effective for Treating and Curing Metabolic Syndrome

Metabolic syndrome is a condition that includes a variety of serious and even fatal symptoms, including:

- Obesity

- High blood pressure

- Elevated blood sugar levels

- Elevated triglyceride levels

- Low DLD cholesterol levels

Metabolic syndrome increases the individual's risk of stroke, heart attack, heart disease, and type two diabetes. However, all symptoms of metabolic syndrome improve drastically while on a low- carb, high- fat diet. Unfortunately, major health organizations continue recommending a low- fat diet for individuals with this condition, even though it does not address the fundamental metabolic issue that causes these serious symptoms.

9. Increasingly Improves the Function of LDL Cholesterol

Low Density Lipoprotein (LDL) is known as the "bad" cholesterol and counter opposite of HDL. This is due to the fact that individuals with higher LDL levels are more likely to suffer from a heart attack. Although this idea goes against what we have been lead to believe about LDL, scientists have found that LDL matters when it comes to our health; not all LDL proteins are equal. This means that the size of the LDL protein particles is important and plays a large role in the state of your health. Individuals whose LDL is mostly made up of small particles have a heightened risk of heart disease, while people with large particles have a lower risk.

It has been found that low- carbohydrate, high- fat diets increase the size of the LDL particles, as well as reduce the number of LDL particles that are flowing through the bloodstream.

10. Low- Carbohydrate Lifestyles Help to Improve Several Brain Disorders

While low- carb diets are beneficial for a number of serious diseases, one of the most valuable uses of sticking to a ketogenic diet is acting as a therapeutic factor for life- altering brain disorders. Glucose is necessary for the brain, however only some parts of the brain are able to burn glucose. This is why your liver will create glucose out of excess protein if you stop consuming carbohydrates. However, a large part of the brain can also utilize ketones; which, as you know, are created when your body's carb consumption is very limited. This amazing and natural function of the ketogenic diet has been practiced for decades to help treat children with epilepsy when medicinal treatment fails.

In a number of cases, the Atkins diet has even cured children of epilepsy. One study concluded that more than half of the children who were fed a low- carb diet had a more than fifty percent reduction in their seizure episodes, with sixteen percent of the kids being cured altogether. The success with the low- carb, high- fat diet in epilepsy patients has inspired doctors and researchers to study the relationship between a ketogenic diet and several other disorders; for example, Parkinson's disease and Alzheimer's disease.

Part 2:

Atkins
21- Day Meal Plan

Chapter 5: 10 No- Carb Breakfast Recipes

1. Bacon, Cheese, and Avocado Breakfast Fiesta

<u>Ingredients</u>

½ of a Medium- Sized Tomato

1 Oz. Water

1 Medium- Sized Spring Onion

1 Slices of Cooked Bacon

1/3 Cup of Shredded Monterey Jack Cheese

½ Small Jalapeno Pepper

2 tsp. of Butter

1 tsp. of Lime Juice

½ Avocado, sliced

½ tsp. of Cilantro

2 Large Eggs

<u>Directions:</u>

1. Start by preparing your homemade salsa. First, chop the tomatoes, spring onion, and jalapeno pepper.

2. Combine these ingredients in bowl with the cilantro and juice from the lime. Set aside for later.

3. In a separate bowl, beat eggs with water. Then, crumble the cooked bacon and set aside.

4. Liquefy the butter at medium heat in a pan. When the pan is coated with the butter, add in half of the egg mixture. Tilt the pan so that the bottom is evenly coated with the egg, then continue cooking until the egg is almost set.

5. Add in the remaining egg, bacon, avocado, and cheese on top of the cooked egg. Let the contents of the pan cook for approximately one minute.

6. Fold the omelet over itself so that the filling is covered. Allow the eggs to cook for another two minutes before removing the omelet from the pan.

7. Serve your omelet with the salsa and enjoy!

2. Baked Eggs and Vegetables

Ingredients

4 Small Asparagus Spears

1 Tbs. of Almond Meal Flour

4 Tbs. of Heavy Whipping Cream

4 tsp. of Parmesan Cheese

2 Large Eggs

A Clove of Garlic, minced

Directions:

1. Heat oven to 400 degrees and prepare a small casserole dish with extra virgin olive oil or baking spray.

2. Next, boil the asparagus for approximately two minutes, until the spears are tender – crisp. Then, drain the vegetables and run them under cold water. Pat the asparagus dry and place in the casserole dish.

3. Pour the heavy cream over top of the asparagus. Now, crack the two eggs on top over the spears.

4. Now, in a bowl, stir the almond flour, cheese, and minced garlic. Sprinkle the mixture over top of the eggs. Put into the oven and bake for six to eight minutes, depending on how you like your eggs.

5. Remove the dish from the oven and enjoy!

3. Ham, Egg, and Garden Vegetable Breakfast Blend

Ingredients

  1 ½ Tbs. of Extra Virgin Olive Oil

  1 Plum Tomato

  2 Tbs. of Butter

  ½ Medium- Sized Onion, chopped

  1 Tbs. of Basil

  1 Medium- Sized Bell Pepper

  2 Oz. of Ham

  3 Large Eggs

  1 Clove of Garlic, minced

Directions:

1. Begin by heating the olive oil in skillet on medium heat. Put the onion into the pan and sauté until they are soft. Next, add in the garlic and cook with the onion for approximately one minute.

2. Next, add the peppers and tomatoes into the skillet. Cover the pan and cook the vegetables for ten minutes, until the veggies have softened. Stir the contents of the pan occasionally.

3. Remove lid from pan and have vegetables to simmer until the sauce thickens, stirring frequently.

4. In a bowl, whisk eggs until blended. Then, in a separate skillet, melt butter to layer the bottom. Add in the eggs and basil, and then cook and scramble the eggs until curds form.

5. Add the vegetable mixture and ham into the eggs and stir the contents until the ingredients are mixed together.

6. Remove your breakfast from the pan and enjoy with salt and pepper!

4. Pepper Rings with Egg Filling

Ingredients

2 Tbs. of Shredded Mozzarella Cheese

½ of a Large Red Bell Pepper

2 tbs. of Extra Virgin Olive Oil

2 Large Eggs

Directions:

1. Slice bell pepper across the middle. Next, cut two 1- inch thick rings from the pepper. Carefully use a knife or spoon to remove the ribs and seeds of the pepper rings.

2. Next, put the pepper rings into a skillet with the extra virgin olive oil. Cook over medium heat.

3. Now, crack one egg into each ring and continue to cook until the egg whites are fully set. Do not flip the egg.

4. Sprinkle the shredded mozzarella cheese onto the eggs and cover the skillet. Allow the cheese to melt for one minute, and then season with salt and pepper. Enjoy!

5. Spicy Eggs and Yogurt

Ingredients

2 Large Eggs

1 Tbs. of Chopped Leek

1 tsp. of Lemon Juice

1/3 Cup of Full Fat Greek Yogurt

4 Tbs. of Chopped Scallion

½ Clove of Garlic, halved

½ tsp. of Oregano

¼ Cup of Spinach

2 Tbs. of Butter, divided

1 ½ Tbs. of Extra Virgin Olive Oil

1 Dash of Chili Powder

Directions:

1. Heat your oven to 300 degrees. Begin by combining the yogurt and garlic in a small bowl. Add in a sprinkle of salt, and then set aside.
2. Add one tablespoon of butter and the oil in a skillet and melt on medium heat. Then, add the scallion and leek into the pan and reduce the heat to a lower setting. Continue

cooking until the ingredients are soft: approximately ten minutes of cooking time.

3. Next, heat to medium – high and add the spinach and lemon juice into the skillet. Cook the spinach until the leaves have wilted, stirring often.

4. Now, transfer the spinach into a separate skillet, leaving the liquid in the original pan. Then, use a spoon to make deep indentations in the middle of the spinach for the eggs.

5. Crack both eggs into each indentation, and then cook until the egg whites have set: approximately ten minutes.

6. In a pan, liquefy the last tablespoon of butter on medium heat. Add in the remaining unused ingredients and cook until the butter begins to foam.

7. Now, remove the garlic from the yogurt dressing and discard. Dollop the yogurt over the eggs and spinach, and serve with a drizzle of spicy butter. Enjoy!

6. New Way for Bacon and Eggs

Ingredients

    1 ½ Oz. of Cream Cheese

    1 Pinch of Thyme

    2 Large Hard- Boiled Eggs

    2 Slices of Bacon

Directions:

1. Heat oven to 400 degrees and coat baking sheet with olive oil spray.

2. Begin preparing the cream cheese filling by combining the thyme and cream cheese in a bowl. Cover filling and put aside for later.

3. Next, peel the hard – boiled eggs, then carefully slice them lengthwise.

4. Use a spoon to remove the yolks from the white halves and discard. Fill two of the egg white halves with the filling, and then use the remaining two to cover the filling.

5. Next, tightly wrap slice of bacon around each of the eggs. Then, place the bacon- wrapped eggs in the baking dish.

6. Bake eggs in oven for thirty minutes. Remove from heat and enjoy!

7. Low- Carb Pancakes

Ingredients

2 Large Eggs

½ tsp. of Cinnamon

2 Oz. of Full Fat Cream Cheese

1 tsp. of Sugar

1 Tbs. of Butter

Directions:

1. Simply combine ingredients with blender; pulse until smooth. Allow the batter to rest for a few minutes as the bubbles settle.

2. Heat the butter in a skillet on medium- high so that it melts as a coating for the bottom of the pan.

3. Next, pour ¼ of the pancake batter into the pan so that it forms the shape of a pancake. Cook until the underside of the pancake is golden brown. Then, flip the cake so that the other side can bake.

4. When the underside has turned golden, remove the pancake from heat and repeat the process until you have used up the rest of the batter. Enjoy!

8. Spinach and Feta Breakfast Quiche

<u>Ingredients</u>

3 Large Eggs

4 Oz. of Button Mushrooms

2 Oz. of Feta Cheese, crumbled

½ Clove of Garlic, minced

5 tsp. of Parmesan Cheese

¼ Cup of Mozzarella Cheese

5 Oz. of Frozen Spinach, thawed

<u>Directions:</u>

1. Heat oven to 350 degrees and prepare a small pie pan with olive oil spray.

2. Start by squeezing the spinach in a paper towel, to remove the excess moisture. Prepare the mushrooms by rinsing them, then thinly slicing them.

3. Place a pan on medium heat, and layer with olive oil spray. Add the mushrooms and garlic into the pan and sauté until mushrooms are soft: approximately 6 minutes.

4. Next, place the spinach into baking dish, followed by the mushrooms. Add the crumbled feta cheese on top of the mushrooms to create a third layer.

5. Beat eggs and parmesan. Then, pour mixture on into the baking dish.

6. Finally, top the quiche with mozzarella cheese, and then put in oven.

7. Bake the quiche for approximately forty minutes, until the top is golden brown. Then, serve and enjoy!

9. Coconut Chia Seed Breakfast Pudding

Ingredients

¼ Cup of Chia Seeds

2 tsp. of Honey

1 Cup of Full Fat Coconut Milk

Directions:

1. Simple combine seeds, honey, and milk in a small bowl. Then, place in the refrigerator overnight.

2. In the morning, remove the bowl from the fridge and enjoy the pudding with a side of your favorite berries.

10. Salmon and Egg Avocados

Ingredients:

2 Large Eggs

1 Avocado

Salt and Pepper

1 Oz. of Smoked Salmon

¼ tsp. of Chili Flakes

Directions:

1. Heat oven to 425 degrees and prepare a sheet with olive oil spray.
2. Slice the avocado in half, lengthwise. Then, remove the seed. Use spoon to remove some of the avocado flesh, so that the holes are big enough for an egg to fit in.
3. Place the avocado halves onto the baking sheet and use the strips of salmon to line the hollows.
4. Crack the eggs into a small bowl, and carefully spoon the yolks and some of the egg whites into the avocado halves.
5. Season your breakfast with spices, and then put in oven. Cook for approximately eighteen minutes.
6. Remove from oven, and then top with the chili flakes. Enjoy!

Chapter 6: 10 Crave- Worthy Lunches

1. Caprese Omega- 3 Salad

<u>Ingredients</u>

¼ Cup of Balsamic Vinegar

½ Cup of Cherry Tomatoes, halved

1 Tbs. of Brown Sugar

2 Oz. of Fresh Mozzarella

4 tsp. of Extra Virgin Olive Oil

1 Avocado, halved, seeded, and diced

2 Cups of Romaine Lettuce, chopped

1 Tbs. of Basil Leaves

1 Boneless, Skinless Chicken Breast, thinly sliced

<u>Directions:</u>

1. Start by preparing the balsamic reduction. Do this by adding the brown sugar and balsamic vinegar into saucepan on medium heat. Allow the sauce to come to a boil, and then lower heat halfway. Cook for approximately seven minutes, and then set aside to cool.

2. Next, in a separate skillet, heat the oil on medium- high heat.

3. Place the chicken breast into the skillet and cook until meat is finished cooking; flipping the chicken once. Allow the chicken to cool before chopping it into cubes.

4. Finally, add the romaine lettuce into a bowl, and add chicken and remaining ingredients. Pour the balsamic vinegar dressing on salad and gently toss. Enjoy!

2. Low- Carb Shrimp Salad

<u>Ingredients</u>

¼ Head of Cauliflower

½ Cucumber

¼ lb. of Raw Shrimp

2 tsp. of Extra Virgin Olive Oil

½ Tbs. of Lemon Zest

1 Tbs. of Chopped Dill

<u>Directions:</u>

1. Preheat your oven to 350 degrees and layer sheet with cooking spray. Begin preparing your salad by peeling and cleaning your shrimp. Additionally, remove the tails as well.

2. Place the shrimp onto the sheet and put into the oven. Cook for eight minutes, until the shrimp is opaque.

3. While the shrimp is cooking, cut the florets off the cauliflower and discard the bottom stalk. Carefully chop the florets into small pieces, then place in a microwave-safe dish.

4. Cook the cauliflower in the microwave for five minutes, so that it is soft, but not mushy.

5. Set aside the shrimp and cauliflower to cool. Then, peel and chop the cucumbers into small pieces.

6. Once cooled, slice the shrimp into halves lengthwise. Then, in a bowl, mix together the all of the ingredients, evenly coating the cauliflower and shrimp with olive oil and lemon juice. Enjoy!

3. Zucchini Protein Pasta

Ingredients

1 Tbs. of Extra Virgin Olive Oil

½ Cup of Cherry Tomatoes

1 Medium Zucchinis

¼ Cup of Sun- Dried Tomatoes

½ Lemon, juiced

½ Cup of Basil, chopped

½ Serving of Vegetable Pasta

1 Oz. of Grated Parmesan Cheese

1 Large Poached Egg

½ Tbs. of Toasted Pine Nuts

Directions:

1. Cook the vegetable pasta in correlation with instructions providing on the packaging. While you are waiting for the pasta to cook, finely dice the cherry tomatoes and transfer them into a bowl.

2. Add the sun- dried tomatoes, garlic, lemon juice, basil, and a sprinkle of red pepper flakes (optional) to the bowl. Then, set the tomato mixture aside and allow to rest for ten minutes.

3. Now, use a spiralizer to spiralize the zucchini to create long noodles that resemble spaghetti. Add the zucchini noodles

and veggie noodles into a deep bowl and toss together with oil.

4. Top your pasta with your homemade tomato sauce and poached egg. Sprinkle parmesan cheese on top with the pine nuts, and enjoy!

4. Portabella Mushroom Burgers

<u>Ingredients</u>

2 Portabella Mushroom Caps, stems removed

1 Slice of Halloumi

1 ½ Tbs. of Balsamic Vinegar

1 Thick Slice of Tomato

1 Tbs. of Extra Virgin Olive Oil

<u>Directions:</u>

1. Heat grill to medium heat, and wash and dry your mushroom caps.

2. In a small shallow dish, use a fork to whisk the balsamic vinegar and extra virgin olive oil. Then, place the mushroom caps gill-side down into to the dressing.

3. Next, place the mushrooms on the grill and cook for approximately five minutes; until they start to sweat. Then, flip the mushrooms so that the other side grills for another three minutes.

4. Place the halloumi on the grill and allow to cook for two minutes on both sides, until the cheese is pliable.

5. Start assembling your burger, using the mushroom caps as the bun and the cheese as the patty. Lightly season the tomato and then place the second mushroom on top to create the sandwich. Enjoy!

5. Spaghetti- Inspired Squash Pasta

Ingredients

     1 Spaghetti Squash

     1 Cup of Kale

     ¾ Cup of Chickpeas, cooked

     2 Cloves of Garlic, min

     1 Tbs. of Extra Virgin Olive Oil

     ½ Cup of Toasted Hazelnuts

     2 Tbs. of Parmesan Cheese

Directions:

1. Heat your oven to 400 degrees, and prepare a sheet with olive oil spray.

2. Begin by slicing your spaghetti squash in half lengthwise, then removing the seeds. Rub each half with half a tablespoon of olive oil on the inside of the vegetable.

3. Place the squash facedown onto sheet and put in oven for forty minutes.

4. As the squash is baking, prepare the filling. Start by washing the kale and removing the ribs of the leaves. Then, roughly chop the leaves into small pieces.

5. In a pan, heat oil and minced garlic for two minutes. Add in the kale and continue cooking until the leaves turn bright green and have just started to wilt.

6. Next, add the chickpeas into the skillet and cook until they are warm. Then, transfer pan from heat and put aside.

7. Remove the baking sheet from the oven and use fork to remove the insides of the squash to form strands of

spaghetti. Transfer the strands into a bowl, and the mix the spaghetti with the kale mixture.

8. Serve your dish topped with hazelnuts and parmesan cheese. Enjoy!

6. Simple Cucumber Salad

<u>Ingredients</u>

1 Medium Cucumber

1 Pinch of Pink Himalayan Salt

2 Tbs. of Rice Vinegar

1 Tbs. of Toasted Sesame Seeds

½ tsp. of Sugar

<u>Directions:</u>

1. Start by peeling the cucumber, and then slicing it in half lengthwise. Next, use a spoon to scrap out the seeds.

2. Use a knife or carefully slice the cucumber into thin slices. Then, use a double layer of paper towels to gently press the excess moisture from the cucumber slices.

3. In a bowl, mix sugar, vinegar, and salt until the sugar is dissolved.

4. In a medium bowl, toss the cucumbers, sesame seeds, and dressing until the mixture is well combined. Enjoy!

7. Broccoli and Feta Salad

<u>Ingredients</u>

1 Cup of Broccoli Florets, finely chopped

3 Tbs. of Feta Cheese

½ Cup of Chickpeas, rinsed

2 Tbs. of Full Fat Yogurt

3 Tbs. of Chopped Red Bell Pepper

½ Tbs. of Lemon Juice

½ Clove of Garlic, minced

Directions:

1. Start by whisking the feta cheese, garlic, and juice from the lemon in a bowl until the mixture is well combined.

2. Next, add the broccoli, red pepper, and chickpeas into the mixture and toss until evenly coated. Enjoy!

8. Tuna Salad with a Twist

Ingredients

6 Oz. of Chunk Tuna, drained and shredded

¼ Cup of Mayonnaise

½ Cup of Canned Artichoke Hearts

1 tsp. of Lemon Juice

2 Tbs. of Chopped Olives

½ tsp. of Oregano

Directions:

1. For this recipe, all you need to do is mix the ingredients together in a bowl. Enjoy!

9. Squash and Cheese Lunch Cakes

<u>Ingredients</u>

2 Cups of Summer Squash, shredded, seeds removed

1 Large Egg

2/3 Cup of Shallots, chopped

1 Tbs. of Extra Virgin Olive Oil

2 tsp. of Chopped Parsley

4 Tbs. of Parmesan Cheese

<u>Directions:</u>

1. Heat oven to 400 degrees. Begin by whisking the egg in a mixing bowl, then adding the shallots, salt, pepper, and parsley to season.

2. Next, place the shredded squash on a kitchen towel and squeeze out any excess liquid. Then, place the squash and cheese into the bowl that contains the egg mixture and combine.

3. Heat oil in skillet on medium heat and place a quarter of the squash batter onto the pan. Gently pat down the squash so that it forms a small cake. Cook the cake until it is brown and toasted. Then, flip the cake and allow to cook until browned.

4. Remove the squash cake form the skillet and repeat with the rest of the batter.

5. Place all of the cakes onto the skillet and carefully transfer into the oven. Bake for approximately eight minutes, and then serve.

10. Simple Chickpea Salad

Ingredients

Ranch Dressing:

1 Shallot, peeled

1 Tbs. of Buttermilk Powder

1 Tbs. of White- Wine Vinegar

½ Tbs. of Dill

¼ Cup of Cottage Cheese

2 Tbs. of Mayonnaise

2 Tbs. of Coconut Milk

Salt and Pepper

Chickpea Salad:

1.5 Cups of Cherry Tomatoes, halved

4 Oz. of Chickpeas, rinsed

8 tsp. of Red Onion, chopped

2 Tbs. of Crumbled Feta Cheese

Directions:

1. Start by preparing the dressing. Place the shallot into food processor and process until thinly chopped. Then, add the mayonnaise, buttermilk, cottage cheese, and vinegar into the processor and process smooth.

2. Pour milk in processor as it is running, along with the salt, pepper, and dill.

3. Now, begin preparing the salad but simply combining all of the salad ingredients in a medium bowl. Drizzle dressing in the bowl with the salad ingredients until evenly coated. Enjoy!

Chapter 7: 10 Simple Weight Loss Dinner Ideas

1. Honey Broiled Salmon

Ingredients

> 1 Scallion, minced
>
> ½ lb. Salmon Fillet, skinned
>
> 1 Tbs. of Honey
>
> 2 tsp. of Soy Sauce
>
> 1 Tbs. of Ginger, minced
>
> 1 Tbs. of Rice Vinegar
>
> 1 Clove of Garlic, minced
>
> ½ tsp. of Toasted Sesame Seeds

Directions:

1. Preheat your broiler and prepare a sheet with olive oil spray.
2. Begin by whisking together the vinegar, ginger, soy sauce, honey, and scallion in a bowl, until the honey has completely dissolved.
3. Next, place the salmon fillet in a sandwich bag and add half of the sauce mixture to marinate the salmon. Seal the plastic bag and place in the refrigerator for fifteen minutes.

4. Once the salmon is finished marinating, place the fillet one to the pan and broil approximately four to six inches away from heat until fully cooked through. This will take about ten minutes.

5. Serve the salmon with a drizzle of the sauce, topped with the sesame seeds. Enjoy!

2. Buffalo Chicken and Artichokes

Ingredients

1 Large Artichoke, trimmed and prepped

¼ Cup of Shredded Cheddar Cheese

1 Lemon, halved

4 Tbs. of Hot Sauce

¼ lbs. of Cooked Ground Chicken

1 ½ Tbs. of Butter

1 Tbs. of Flour

½ Cup of Coconut Milk

Directions:

1. Begin by bringing pot of water to boil. Then, add the artichoke and lemon to the water, and bring to simmer. Cover pot and let cook for thirty minutes.

2. When the artichoke is finished cooking, transfer from the pot to a kitchen towel to allow the water to drain.

3. Now, preheat your oven to 400 degrees and prepare sheet with spray. Place the artichokes onto the sheet and splay the leaves.

4. Use a spoon to add the ground chicken in between the artichoke layers.

5. Next, liquefy butter in saucepan on medium heat. Add flour and beat with the butter for one minute. In small amount, pour the coconut milk into the saucepan, whisking the mixture until thickened.

6. Remove the saucepan from the stovetop and stir in the hot sauce and cheese.

7. Carefully pour the cheese over top of the artichokes and put in oven for ten minutes. Remove from oven and enjoy!

3. Simple Taco Skillet

Ingredients

½ lb. of Ground Beef

1 Cup of Baby Kale

½ Yellow Onion, diced

Taco Seasoning

1 Bell Pepper, diced

½ Cup of Shredded Cheddar Cheese

½ Can of Diced Tomatoes with Chilies

1 Zucchini, diced

Directions:

1. In a medium pan, brown the beef and crumble. Then, drain the excess grease.

2. Next, add the peppers and onion into the skillet and continue cooking until both vegetables have browned. Then, add in the canned tomatoes, taco seasoning, and as much water as the seasoning packet instructions calls for.

3. Now, add the kale into the taco beef mixture and mix well. Add in the cheese and allow it to melt into the beef, stirring frequently. Once the cheese has melted, remove from heat and enjoy over a bowl of lettuce.

4. Spinach and Artichoke Frittata

<u>Ingredients</u>

3 Large Eggs

1 Shallot, diced

2 Oz. of Marinated Artichokes, diced

1 Tbs. of Extra Virgin Olive Oil

1 Clove of Garlic, minced

4 Broccoli Florets, chopped fine

1 Tbs. of Chives

½ Cup of Spinach

1 Green Onion, finely sliced

2 Tbs. of Feta Cheese

Directions:

1. Coat a skillet with the oil on medium- heat. Add the shallots and garlic into the pan, and sauté for two minutes.

2. Next, add the broccoli into the pan and continue cooking until soft. Then, add in the spinach and stir into the mixture until the leaves have wilted.

3. While the vegetables are cooking, whisk the eggs and chives together in a mixing bowl. Pour the eggs into the vegetables and stir together.

4. Now, add in the artichoke hearts and allow the frittata to cook until the eggs are almost set. Preheat your broiler to 500 degrees.

5. Reduce the heat of the stovetop to medium/ low and continue cooking for an another two minutes. Transfer the skillet to the oven and broil until the frittata is browned.

6. Serve your dinner with crumbled feta cheese and enjoy!

5. Enchilada Zucchini Boats

Ingredients

Sauce:

½ Garlic Clove

¼ Cup of Chicken Broth

½ Tbs. of Hot Sauce

Salt and Pepper

1/3 Cup of Tomato Sauce

A Pinch of Chili Powder and Ground Cumin

Zucchini Boats:

1 Zucchini

¼ Cup of Green Bell Pepper, diced

½ tsp. of Extra Virgin Olive Oil

2 Tbs. of Chopped Cilantro

¼ Cup of Green Onions, diced

1 ½ Tbs. of Water

4 Oz. of Cooked Chicken Breast, shredded

½ Tbs. of Tomato Paste

½ Clove of Garlic, crushed

A Pinch of Cumin, Oregano, and Chili Powder

¼ Cup of Shredded Cheddar Cheese

Directions:

1. For the sauce, coat a saucepan with cooking spray and sauté the garlic. Then, add in the chili powder, broth, tomato sauce, and cumin to the pan and bring to a boil.

2. Reduce heat and let sauce to simmer for about ten minutes. Then, set aside to use later.

3. Now, bring pot of water to boil and preheat your oven to 400 degrees. Prepare a baking dish with cooking spray.

4. Slice the zucchini in half lengthwise and use a spoon to scoop out the inside, so that the shell is ¼ inch thick. Roughly chop the removed flesh and transfer into a small bowl.

5. Place the zucchini halves into the boiling water. Cook the zucchini for one minute, and then carefully remove the halves from the pot.

6. In a skillet, heat oil on medium- low heat. Add the onion, pepper, and garlic into the pan and cook until the onions are translucent.

7. Next, add the zucchini flesh into the skillet with the cilantro, and cook for approximately four minutes. Add the spices, water, and tomato paste into the pan and cook for three more minutes.

8. Now, add the chicken to the skillet and mix with the contents of the pan for a few minutes.

9. Pour half of the enchilada sauce into the baking dish, and then place the zucchini halves onto the dish, with the cut side facing up.

10. Fill the hollowed inside of the zucchinis with the chicken mixture, pressing the meat into the vegetable until filled. Use the rest of the sauce to cover the filled zucchini halves, and then top with cheddar cheese.

11. Cover the baking dish with aluminum foil and place in the oven. Allow to bake for thirty minutes, and serve once the zucchini is cooked through.

6. Pizza Frittata

Ingredients

½ tsp. of Oregano

6 Large Eggs

3 Tbs. of Dry Red Wine

3 Tbs. of Extra Virgin Olive Oil

½ Cup of Half- and Half

½ Cup of Crushed Tomatoes

1 Cup of Hot Pepperoni, chopped

¼ Cup of Parmesan Cheese

3 Oz. of Shredded Mozzarella Cheese

1 Clove of Garlic, chopped

1 tsp. of Hot Sauce

1 Tbs. of Grated Onion

1 tsp. of Chopped Parsley

Directions:

1. Heat oven to 400 degrees. Begin by whisking the eggs, cream, hot sauce, and parmesan cheese in a bowl.
2. Next, heat ½ of the oil in a pan on medium- high heat. Add the eggs into the pan and move them frequently until they start to firm.
3. Place the skillet into the oven and bake for approximately seven minutes.

4. In a separate skillet, heat remaining oil on medium- high heat and add cook the garlic, onion, and oregano for three minutes. Pour the wine into the pan and slightly reduce the heat.

5. Add the tomatoes into the skillet and simmer for ten minutes, until the sauce has thickened.

6. Remove the skillet from the oven and pour the tomato sauce over top. Sprinkle with mozzarella cheese and place into the oven once again for ten minutes. Top your frittata with parsley and enjoy!

7. Classic Chicken Wings

<u>Ingredients</u>

1 lb. of Wings and Drumettes

½ Tbs. of Butter

1 Tbs. of Thyme

3 Garlic Cloves, crushed

¼ Cup of Hot Sauce

For Dip:

½ Cup of Greek Yogurt

¼ Cup of Blue Cheese Crumbles

<u>Directions:</u>

1. Heat oven to 375 degrees and prepare a baking sheet with cooking spray.

2. In a medium bowl, season the chicken with salt and pepper.

3. Over low heat, melt butter in pan. Add in the garlic and thyme, and let simmer for two minutes. Then, add in the hot sauce, stirring the ingredients together.

4. Pour the hot sauce mixture over the chicken and toss well to evenly coat. Let the wings marinate in the refrigerator for a half hour.

5. While the wings are marinating, begin making your dressing. Simply combine the blue cheese and yogurt together in a bowl, and refrigerate for later.

6. Place the wings and drummettes onto the baking sheet and transfer to the oven. Bake for thirty minutes. Turn the chicken over, and baste with more hot sauce. Then, bake for an additional twenty- five minutes.

7. Remove wings from oven and let to cool before serving with the blue cheese dip. Enjoy!

8. Easy Steak Rolls

Ingredients

½ lb. of Flank Steak

½ Cup of Green Beans

¼ Cup of Steak Marinade

¼ White Onion, sliced into strips

½ Red Bell Pepper, sliced into strips

1 Tbs. of Extra Virgin Olive Oil

Directions:

1. First, marinade your steak in a plastic sandwich bag for thirty minutes with the steak marinade. While your steak is marinating, preheat your oven to 350 degrees and prepare a baking sheet with cooking spray.

2. Next, heat a skillet over medium heat and heat the olive oil in the pan.

3. Slice the steaks in halves. Take a little bit of the peppers, green beans, and onion slices, and tightly wrap the steak slices around the vegetables. Use toothpicks to secure the wrap.

4. Now, add the steak rolls to the skillet and sear for one minute on all sides of the wrap.

5. Carefully transfer the steak rolls onto the baking sheet and place in the oven. Cook for ten minutes, and then remove from the oven. Enjoy!

9. Simple Stuffed Chicken

Ingredients

1 Boneless, Skinless Chicken Breast

2 Oz. of Fresh Mozzarella, sliced

3 Oz. of Roasted Red Peppers, sliced into small pieces

2 Basil Leaves

2 Tbs. of Parmesan Cheese

½ Tbs. of Italian Dressing

Directions:

1. Heat oven to 400 degrees, and prepare a baking dish with cooking spray.

2. Use a knife to butterfly the chicken, cutting the breast lengthwise with about ¼ of an inch from the other side.

3. Spread the chicken breast into the dish, so that you can stuff it. Use salt and pepper to season the chicken.

4. Simply layer the roasted red pepper, and mozzarella cheese onto one side of the chicken. Carefully fold the other half over top, tucking in the stuffed ingredients snuggly into the chicken.

5. Drizzling the Italian dressing over top of the chicken, then place the dish into the oven. Bake for thirty to thirty- five minutes, until the chicken is full cooked.

6. Remove chicken from oven, and turn on your broiler to a high setting. Add any remaining mozzarella cheese and parmesan cheese onto the chicken and place into the oven once more.

7. Broil until the cheese turned golden brown, then remove from heat. Enjoy!

10. Cauliflower Rice

<u>Ingredients</u>

1 Cup of Cauliflower

2 tsp. of Soy Sauce

¼ Cup of Onion, chopped

¼ Cup of Baby Carrots, chopped

1 Tbs. of Extra Virgin Olive Oil

¼ Cup of Thawed Frozen Peas

1 Egg, beaten lightly

1 Green Onion, chopped

½ tsp. of Sesame Oil

½ Cup of Bean Sprouts

Directions:

1. Slice the bottom of the cauliflower off, and then cut the cauliflower into florets. Dry off excess water.

2. Place the florets into a food processor and pulse until you achieve the consistency of rice.

3. Next, heat half of oil in skillet on medium- high heat. Add in the onion and fry until it is light brown. Transfer the onions into a bowl and set aside for later.

4. In a small mixing bowl, whisk the egg with the sesame oil and soy sauce. Add a bit more olive oil into the skillet, then quickly scramble the eggs.

5. Transfer the scrambled eggs from the skillet to the bowl with the onion.

6. Add the rest of the olive oil into the skillet and place the cauliflower, green onions, carrots, bean sprouts, and peas in the pan. Stir fry the ingredients for three minutes, then reduce to a lower heat setting.

7. Add in more soy sauce if desired, then cover until the cauliflower is good all the way through. Add the egg and cooked onions into the skillet once more and allow the ingredients to cook together for two minutes.

8. Serve and enjoy!

Conclusion

I hope this book was able to help you to understand the Atkins diet, as well as feel inspired to begin the first phase right now!

The next step is to make the decision to create a better life for yourself by changing your eating habits. You can have the body of your dreams and the greatest health you are able to achieve just by following this intensive meal plan. Health is the most valuable gift you could ever give yourself.

Finally, if you enjoyed this book, please take the time to share your thoughts and post a review on Amazon. It'd be greatly appreciated!

Thank you and good luck!